Bioresonance Therapy

Healing with the body's own oscillations and with the oscillations of substances

by

Reinhold D. Will

Jopp-Verlag

1, 2, 3, 4, 5 edition 2000, 1999, 1998

Translator. Dr Bojan Jagodic, Dublin
Editor: Christine Lawrie, Shrewsbury
Cover design: Kreativ Design Gerd Aumann, Wiesbaden
Graphics: Regumed-Institut, Gräfelfing
Production: Druckerei Fritz Steinmeier, Nördlingen
Printed in Germany

ISBN 3-89698-114-5

Contents

Preface: He feels like a new person now. . .

N.R., 18 years of age, spent three and a half weeks in a dermatological hospital until he was discharged as being "incurably ill". The diagnosis did not extend further than the vague "suspicion of psoriasis, possibly acne rosea". Therapeutically, the whole spectrum of the usual treatments was applied: from radiation through cortisone to saltwater baths. However, 99 % of the diet he was supposed to follow consisted of foods to which he had an allergic reaction. So it is no small wonder that he could not be cured and that he actually felt worse after his time in hospital. When this young man finally came to the bioresonance surgery he was a sorry sight. Almost his whole body was covered in hard scales, while beneath them the skin was red and infected. Because of the itching, he constantly had the urge to scratch himself which immediately led to new infections that spread rapidly. His scalp, in particular, was covered in thick scales and it was impossible to remove them.

Disfigured like this, the youngster hardly dared to leave home, did not attend school any more and isolated himself completely. Nobody was allowed to visit him and he was terribly ashamed of his appearance. His bad overall condition also affected his sleeping-waking rhythm so that he was only able to sleep for short periods.

In taking his history it became apparent that there was an allergic disposition in the family. His mother was inclined to have allergic reactions and his brother had a minor case of psoriasis. And indeed, tests with bioresonance treatment showed that the patient suffered from a multitude of allergies. Additionally, toxic stresses, for instance from pesticides with which he had been in contact during a holiday job in a garden centre, worsened his clinical picture.

A clinical picture this severe requires a very specific approach in bioresonance treatment. After in-depth tests, a treatment plan was devised that would gradually bring relief to the patient from his allergies and toxins and restore his skin to normal. A central point was the treatment of

the allergies, because the patient reacted allergically to nearly everything that constitutes the daily diet: cow's milk, milk sugar (lactose), sugar, wheat, buckwheat, rye, oats, barley, corn, yeast, apples, carrots, egg white, nuts and herbs. He also reacted to pollen, sheep's wool, down, guinea pigs, horses, nickel and cobalt. In such severe cases, an allergic reaction to moulds (fungi) often plays a role as well, and this patient suffered from a candida allergy which also had to be treated.
The toxic stresses that had to be removed with the help of the BICOM device were polychloridated biphenyls (PCBs), chloridated carbohydrates, formaldehyde, DDT, lead, cadmium and carbendazin. (The BICOM device is a device with which to carry out the bioresonance therapy; BICOM is an abbreviation of BIo-COMmunication which means that body and device are communicating with each other). Also, the scar from his appendectomy proved to be an interference field that had to be eliminated with bioresonance therapy.
A big problem was his complete reaction rigidity. In the bioresonance therapy, therefore, the first aim was to restore the patient's ability to react, which took a few weeks. The real treatment could only be started after this had been achieved.
The treatment consisted of eliminating the allergies, excreting the toxins from the system and supporting measures to balance out the general energetic situation. Additionally the patient was given medication to improve his metabolism as well as vitamins, folic acid and an iron preparation based on an examination of his blood. The skin was treated with skin-fungus and skincare ointments. And of course our youngster had to abstain from the allergising foods during the treatment.
This book will tell you how a bioresonance practitioner approaches an illness, which circumstances he has to pay attention to and how he treats them. You will find out why an illness has to be treated in a holistic way and how this is possible in the framework of bioresonance therapy. And finally you will find out why bioresonance therapy is as successful as it is.
With the patient described above, bioresonance therapy was more successful than anyone could have hoped for. Today, he is completely cured from his illness. He no longer has any scales. He went back to school, visits his friends and once again is the happy youngster he used to be before the illness struck him.

The reason why treatments are successful

Successful treatments go into resonance with the patient's own oscillations

Conventional medicine applies treatments on the basis of its diagnosis ("inflammatory arthritis of the joints", "acute gastritis", "chronic inflammation of the renal pelvis", etc.), that are supposed to be helpful for everyone who falls victim to the condition. But every person is an individual and different from anybody else.

The same thing is valid for illnesses: every illness is individual. For that reason the treatment cannot consist of standardised therapies but has to address the personal particularities of the patients.

Every illness is individual

This means: the treatment has to be adapted precisely to the particular patient. Put in the modern terminology: the treatment has to be able to "go into resonance" with him.

Therapeutic impulses have to be in resonance

But what is the meaning of the expression "go into resonance"?

As we all know, the human being, like animals and plants, is living matter. We are familiar with this matter as being a solid substance that we can touch, measure and weigh.

Matter is compressed energy

The scientists of quantum theory recognised ninety years ago that matter is nothing but compressed energy.

Max Planck

The famous physicist Max Planck (1858–1947) said: ". . . after my research into the atom I can tell you this: strictly speaking there is no matter. All matter only develops and exists through a force, which brings the atom particles into oscillation and bonds them into the minute solar system of the atom. Matter *per se* does not exist, there is only the invigorating, invisible, immortal spirit as the primeval foundation of matter. . . ."

Albert Einstein

And the physicist Albert Einstein (1879–1955) deliberated: "We can therefore consider matter as that area of space in which the field is extremely dense ... In this new physics there is no room for both field and matter, because the field is the only reality."

Why is this important for medical science?

Why do we have to grapple with the fact that in reality matter is compressed energy?

Why do we have to be disturbed by the fact that our conventional scientific picture of the human being – the one that is at the basis of conventional medicine – is not correct?

Only the adoption of new knowledge will lead us to new medical successes

Very simple: because only the adoption of new knowledge can lead us to new medical successes. Only this step forward can lead us out of the present medical cul-de-sac.

It does not help to deny the facts, to defend obsolete knowledge, or to denigrate or fight the new knowledge; new times require new ways of thinking and acting.

The body is matter as well as energy

The new medicine – still apostrophised as *alternative medicine* – incorporates the fact that the human body consists of energy-matter and is animated by energy. It is regulated and controlled by information. All its functions run materially but are regulated and controlled by information – beginning with our metabolism up to the perpetuation of the different physical "balances" such as electrolyte balance, water balance, acid-base balance.

> For this reason the new medicine is a medicine of matter, energy and information.

Matter, energy and information are of equal importance

In it, all three of them have an equal place: on the level of matter, the biochemical processes are dealt with in diagnosis and treatment; on the energetic level, biophysical processes are involved; and on the informational level, bio-cybernetic processes are considered.

Examples

An example: somebody who has to carry a weight to the second floor of a house needs a body (= matter) with which he can carry the weight, he needs power (= energy) to carry it and he needs to know where to carry it to (= information).
Another example: a physical immune system that has to fight an allergen needs material antibodies, energy for the biochemical processes of the defence and information on which substances to defend against and in what way.

Resonance

Bioresonance

A principle called resonance plays a central role in regulating and controlling these processes. However, in medicine this principle is called bioresonance because it is concerned with living organisms.

What is resonance or bioresonance?

You probably already know the term "resonance". It stems from Latin and means "resound, echo", also "resonate". What is resounding, what is echoing, what is resonating? If a singer hits a note a tuning fork will resound, or resonate, if he sings the exact note for which the tuning fork is calibrated. So if he holds a tuning fork in his hand that has been calibrated to the note "g", then he has to sing the note "g" to make it resonate with his voice, otherwise it will not. If he does, it goes into resonance with the voice of the singer, or the voice of the singer with the tuning fork.

The oscillation image of the transmitter has to be identical to that of the receiver

This means: to develop a resonance, the oscillation image of the transmitter has to be identical to that of the receiver. A human body in medicine can only resonate with a transmitted signal if it is receptive to that signal; in other words, if the signal has the same frequency as the body.

> Healing impulses can only make the body resonate optimally if they correspond with its own frequency.

A therapeutic impulse has to go into resonance with the body in a specific way

Only when a therapeutic impulse goes into resonance with the human body in a specific way is it possible for it to have the intended healing effect. That is the principle of bioresonance. If it does not go into resonance then the healing will only be accidental.

> Bioresonance is the central principle of healing processes. For that reason bioresonance is the key to becoming healthy.

The resonance principle limits the receptivity of the patient for therapeutic impulses to a certain spectrum of oscillation frequencies. Correspondingly, the central finding of bioresonance research is:

> A therapeutic impulse can only have the intended effect if it can go into resonance (bioresonance) with the organism.

Prof. Dr. Cyril W. Smith from Salford University in England discovered that therapeutic impulses that go exactly into resonance with the organism can have an effect even after a very short effective time (in fragments of a second). Therapeutic impulses that barely, or do not at all, go into resonance only have an effect after a relatively long effective time (after several minutes).

Prof. Dr. W.R. Adey from the University of California in the USA confirmed that therapeutic impulses have to address the individual frequencies and also that the strength of the impulses has to be in the individual areas to be certain to have an effect. It is not a case of "a lot helps a lot". An impulse has to be exactly in the amplitude spectrum to be able to have the intended effect without side-effects.

The oscillation of allergens, pesticides etc. can also

be brought into resonance with their own oscillations that have been previously stored in the body. This is the case for instance, if an allergic reaction is triggered, or when the practitioner is testing if the oscillation of a certain allergen has already been stored in the body, or when allergen oscillations have to be eliminated from the body. I will treat this subject in depth in the section on allergic illnesses. (See page 64.)

Resonance is also necessary in oscillations of substances

Of course we should not ignore the fact that health, illness and healing also have their individual and psychological aspects. Accordingly, attention has to be given to these aspects in the treatment.

Successful treatments take environmental factors into account

A big problem of our time is the fact that environmental factors put stresses on the human defence system. This should not be ignored by any practitioner. Toxins and pesticides in the air and in substances, electromagnetic oscillations both indoors and out, heavy metals in the body etc. are slowly but surely overwhelming our defence systems. They put us under such great stress that in more and more cases they lead to faulty controls. The increase in the number of allergic reactions is an example that speaks for itself.

Consider environmental factors in diagnosis and treatment

The application of the bioresonance principle

The way bioresonance therapy using BICOM technology works

Scientists have proven: our whole infinite universe is a "sea of energy" in which solid bodies called stars and planets have been formed through compression of this energy.

One of these bodies of compressed energy is our Earth. Naturally, not only the Earth is compressed energy but also everything material on it, including human beings. Albert Einstein showed the equality of matter and energy in his famous formula: $E=MC^2$.

The human body is an electromagnetic field

This means that the human body, as compressed energy, is an electromagnetic field. Depending on the nature of the examination, this field presents itself either as electromagnetic particles (corpuscles) or as electromagnetic waves (oscillations). This finding is of utmost importance for medicine: with it a breakthrough to a totally new dimension has been achieved – energetic medicine.

Energetic medicine

New diagnostic and therapeutic possibilities in new medicine

This means that in diagnosis and treatment the body can be examined and treated from its energetic side. Consequently, new medicine has entered a new area that opens up new diagnostic and therapeutic possibilities (while conventional medicine still stays on the materialistic level and rejects everything else as "unscientific"). Bioresonance is one of the new medical disciplines (methods) based on this new scientific knowledge that could be developed from these new findings. It works with the electromagnetic oscillations of patients and of substances.

Franz Morell, M.D.

The German doctor Franz Morell, M.D. is the "father" of bioresonance treatment. He worked successfully for years with electro-acupuncture. One day in 1977, on the basis of his experience in electro-acupuncture, he had the brilliant idea that maybe his treatments could become even more accurate if he used the oscillations of his patients instead of those of medication. To realise this idea he had an electronic device built that could receive and return the body oscillations of his patients via electrodes.

New successes in treatment with bioresonance therapy

He modified these oscillations in the device according to certain programs that were especially developed for this purpose. The results were stunningly successful. Dr. Morell could influence illnesses with his new method that could hardly be treated any other way.

MORA treatment

In this way, Dr. Morell founded one of the most exact treatment procedures in medicine available at present. Initially it was called "MORA" treatment after the discoverer, F. Morell, and the engineer who had made the device, E. Rasche. Years later, Hans Brügemann of the Brügemann Institute (this Institute has since changed its name to Regumed – Institute for Regulatory Medicine) called it "bioresonance therapy" because this describes the working principle better and for reasons of copyright protection.

These days, there are several producers of devices for bioresonance therapy. They differ enormously in design, maintenance and use. To avoid confusion, I will only discuss bioresonance therapy with the BICOM device and will ignore the differing use of other versions.

The human being is a transmitter and receiver of electromagnetic oscillations

Bioresonance therapy takes as its starting point the fact that the human body – being an energy field – can transmit and receive electromagnetic oscillations.

We experience some people having a "magnetism" differing from our own. This can be pleasant or unpleasant depending on the effect it has on us. Having read something about resonance, you now know that this is a resonance phenomenon.

The oscillations can be used for diagnosis

In bioresonance therapy, the transmission and reception of electromagnetic oscillations is used to diagnose the energetic situation of the patient as well as for testing medication etc. and treatment. We will describe how this is done later.

The energy patterns of the body can be altered

But the energy patterns of the body can also be altered. This can happen, for instance, through illness or the effect of radiation. In fact, every influence on the body changes its energy field, be it energies that are favourable for the body or be it energies that are disadvantageous. However, most factors can have an advantageous as well as a disadvantageous effect, depending on dosage and nature. Just consider the life-giving sunlight that can burn the skin when over exposed, or medication which although it has a healing effect can at the same time have side-effects, or foods that give us energy but can also trigger allergic reactions.

Oscillations can be bundled and transmitted

Oscillations spread in space in a range depending on their intensity. They can be fed through cables as well as transmitted through radio signals. Bioresonance therapy uses both possibilities in taking the oscillations of patients and substances through electrodes, and feeding them via a cable or infra-red transmitter to the therapy device. In reverse, the device can transmit back therapeutic oscillations of the patient, or of substances like allergens, medicines etc. through cables and electrodes to the patient.

> Bioresonance therapy is a therapy that uses electromagnetic oscillations.

The human body emits different oscillations: cells, tissues and organs each have their specific oscillations.

Individual oscillation image

These individual oscillations are connected to each other and have a mutual influence. Together they form the total oscillation spectrum of the patient – the individual oscillation image.

You can imagine that the oscillations of a healthy person are structured differently to the oscillations of a sick person. The oscillations of a healthy person are harmonious and free of the distortions that you will find in the disharmonious oscillations of a sick person. In sick people, the oscillation of foreign substances like amalgam, bacteria and pesticides that are stored in the body, interfere with the oscillation image. Sick organs also do not oscillate harmoniously. The individual oscillation image informs us about the health or illness of the patient and it can give the decisive clue for an exact diagnosis and the appropriate treatment!

In sick people the oscillations of foreign substances interfere with the oscillation image

Oscillations of the body disclose health and illness

In medicine, the harmonious oscillations are called physiological oscillations because they are emitted from healthy, functioning organs. But they also give information about a well-functioning, self-healing power of the body. The disharmonious oscillations are called pathogenic or pathologic oscillations depending on whether sickening oscillations (for instance, of amalgam) or sick oscillations (for instance, of a sick kidney) are concerned.

Physiological oscillations

Pathogenic or pathologic oscillations

> Your health and your illness are expressed in your personal oscillation image.

The following picture (page 20) shows the difference of the oscillations. The harmonious oscillations (middle curve) flow uninterrupted as in a sine curve. If the disharmonious oscillations (bottom curve) supersede these oscillations, we get the top picture that shows the distorted oscillation image.

The oscillations shown are only a model. In reality the oscillations are much more complex. Also, there are no harmonious oscillations as depicted because nobody is really completely healthy.

Initially, bioresonance therapy, based on Dr. Morell's original idea, was a treatment with the patient's own oscillations. But because he developed bioresonance therapy from electro-acupuncture he soon included medicines; in other words, the oscillations of substances were added to the patient's own oscillations.

Patient's own oscillations

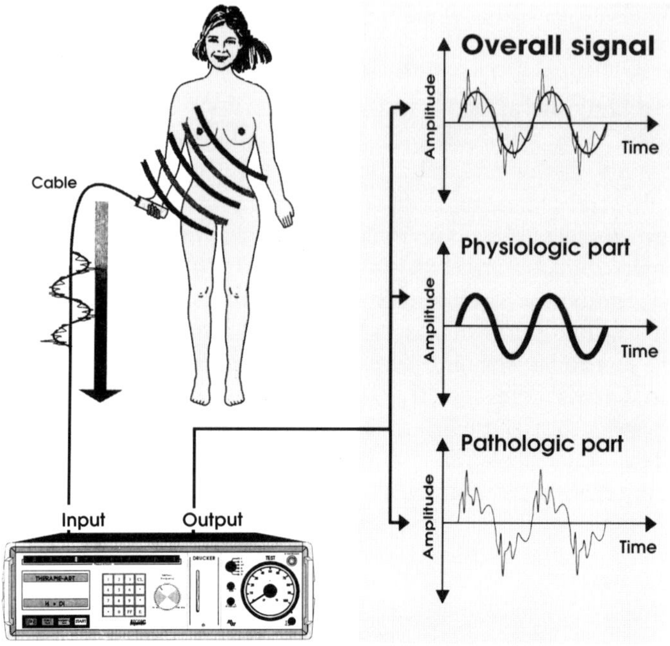

With the help of a separator the physiologic (harmonious) and pathologic (disharmonious) oscillations can be separated and specifically treated.

Oscillations from substances

As time went by, bioresonance practitioners found that it is also possible to diagnose and treat problems with the oscillations of other substances. As an example: it can be used to find out which substances the patient has an allergic reaction to, or it can establish whether childhood illnesses that have been suppressed with antibiotics are still a serious stress for the body.

Bioresonance therapy is a treatment with electromagnetic oscillations of *patients and substances.*

If the disharmonious oscillations are to be remedied in bioresonance therapy, which is an important goal as I will describe later, then the question remains: how can this be done?

Inverted oscillation

Dr. Morell found the answer to this question as well: by giving them to the patient in a turned-around mirror-image way, or "inverted". He got this idea when he remembered a physical law that says that oscillations are influenced by their exact mirror-image. Dr. Morell was the first to apply this law in medicine.

Relief of the body's defence by inverting disharmonious oscillations

The effect: disharmonious oscillations of the patient are diminished or even eliminated by their inversion (mirror-image switching). The stressed regulatory force thus gains relief from them. With this method it is possible to treat disharmonious oscillations of the patient and the oscillations of foreign substances (e.g. pesticides) that are stored in the body depending on whether the patient's own inverted oscillations are used or those of the foreign substances.

Specific elimination of pathologic oscillations

By inverting oscillations, a breakthrough was reached in medicine that previously could not have been imagined, namely the specific relief of the body's own regulatory systems from stressing oscillations.

Bioresonance, oscillations of patients and substances, distinction between harmonious and disharmonious oscillation, inversion of disharmonious oscillation – they all realise the ideal of an individual treatment.

But there was still one problem: as in homeopathy, notwithstanding the individual control of the therapy impulses, there was still too much "initial deterioration".

The problem was solved by a further development of the treatment device by Hans Brügemann: he introduced the attenuation of therapy impulses. This means that bioresonance therapy using BICOM technology can now be adapted to the individual sensitivity of over-sensitive patients and small children, an improvement that fulfils the precision of the intensity of the treatment as demanded by Prof. Adey.

Better treatment effect by attenuation or amplification of the therapeutic impulse

By attenuation or amplification of therapeutic impulses with the BICOM technology, the treatment is more precise and more effective.

How does bioresonance therapy work?

Oscillations control physical processes

As we know from physics, electromagnetic oscillations are information carriers as well as information in themselves. They can control engines and living beings on the basis of their specific characteristics.
Just imagine you get a postcard from the post office that you can come and pick up a new directory. You react by going to the post office to collect a directory. Thus you react to an information with an act. The postcard was the information carrier and the message that the directory was ready to be collected was the information.
In medicine it is similar. A tablet or the water, or alcohol, solution of a medicine is the information carrier; the therapeutic information it contains triggers the biochemical processes. The body's own energy takes care of the effect of the medicine. Bioresonance treatment uses electromagnetic oscillations to trigger biochemical processes in the sense of healing with the information they contain.

> Bioresonance therapy controls the healing processes through information.

Front view

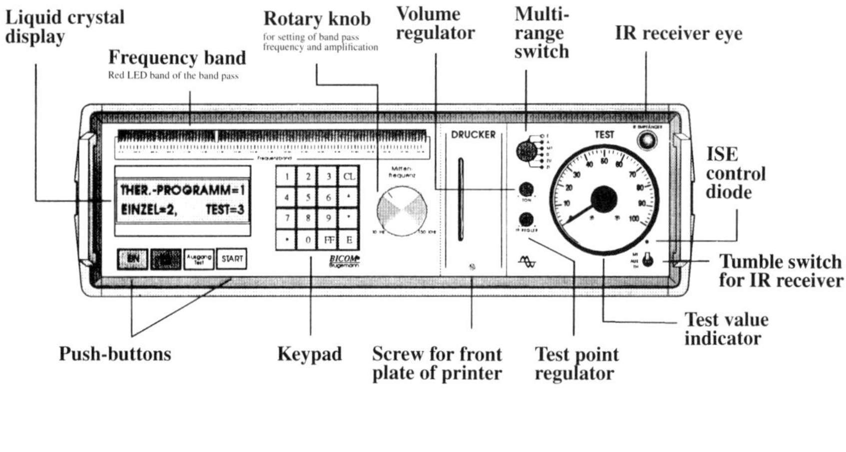

Treatment with the BICOM therapy device

Bioresonance treatment using BICOM technology is applied with the BICOM therapy device. This device consists of three parts: the therapy part (left on the drawing on page 22), the printer (centre) and the test part (right).

Energetic diagnosis by measurement of acupuncture points

The centrepiece of the bioresonance diagnosis is the energetic diagnosis. The patient holds a cylinder electrode in his or her hand and the practitioner measures the skin resistance of certain points (acupuncture points) with a test stylus, for instance on the tips of fingers and toes.

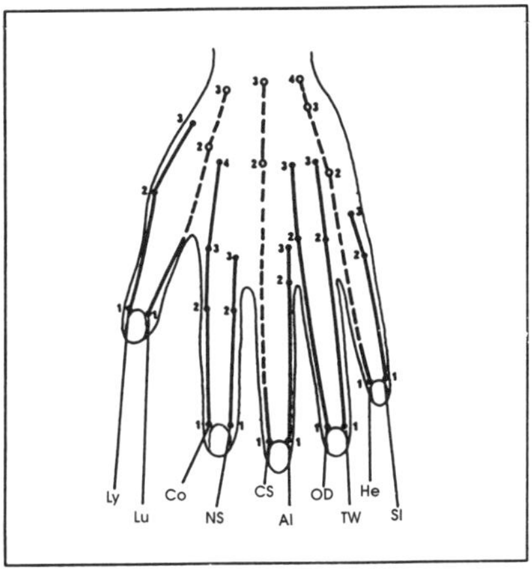

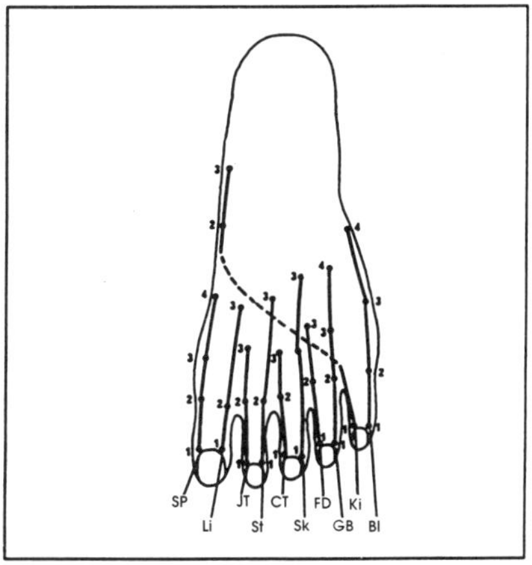

The values of the test that shows the energetic content of the measured meridians can be read from the round scale of the test part (on the right hand side of the picture on page 22). The division of the scale is from 0 to 100. The meaning of the reading will be explained in the next chapter.

The probable effect of a medicine can be tested

This scale also shows the values that are reached in testing medicines. If the indicator goes towards 50 in the test, in comparison to the value previously tested

without the medicine, then the medicine can be applied in the treatment with a probability of success.
In treatment with the BICOM device the patient is again connected to the device via electrodes. In the basic treatment that is aimed at improving the overall energy of the body itself, the patient gives his body's own energy to the device through electrodes/cable. He gets oscillations back through cable/electrodes after they have been subjected to an adaptation in the device corresponding to the specific illness.
In the follow-up treatments, in which for instance the inverted oscillations of an allergen are modulated on the patient, the allergen is put into an aluminium or brass beaker from which the oscillations of the allergen are fed into the BICOM therapy device. From there they are passed to the patient through the cable/ electrodes after they have been adapted (modification). The displays that play a role in this process have been grouped on the left-hand side of the device. The therapy program or the individual parameter that the practitioner has set can be read in the liquid crystal display. Depending on the specific illness the practitioner can either use tested, stored treatment programs or put together an individual program on the basis of tests on the patients.

Individual setting of treatment parameters

The most important individual settings are:

- Type of treatment: in the treatment, harmonious as well as disharmonious oscillations can be used, as described before. The liquid crystal display shows which type of oscillation has been chosen.
- Amplification: the oscillations that have been chosen have to be amplified or attenuated in line with the patient's ability to react and the therapeutic effect intended.
- Treatment time: the therapeutic effect also depends on the effective time of the therapeutic impulse.

The practitioner enters the code numbers for the setting of therapy programs and individual settings on the keypad on the right-hand side, beside the liquid crystal display.
As you have read, the BICOM device works with the

patient's own oscillation or those of substances. A red cursor moves in the frequency band in the therapy part above the liquid crystal display when these oscillations in the different frequency areas are transmitted to the patient. The speed with which the cursor moves up and down indicates the speed at which these oscillations are sequentially taken up and transmitted to the patient. If the practitioner only wants to use one single frequency he can set this with the rotary knob on the right-hand side of the therapy section. The cursor will then remain static on the corresponding point of the frequency band.

Fine tuning of therapeutic signals

With the printer in the middle of the device, the practitioner can print out the code of the pre-set programs and the individual settings as well as the results of the tests and put them in the patient's file for documentation. On the basis of these print-outs he can follow the progress of the treatment.

Documentation of data in diagnosis and treatment

The practice of bioresonance therapy using BICOM technology

The start of a successful treatment is an exact diagnosis. A commonplace? Sure, but how often is it followed? In any case, it is of particular importance in the bioresonance treatments. Without an exact knowledge of the causes of the illness, the bioresonance practitioner can get some results just applying the basic therapies, but he will not be able to fully use all the possibilities of the procedure. Just remember: one of the most important findings of the new medicine is the fact that has already been discussed in the first chapter – that a real success in treatment can only be expected if the treatment corresponds very precisely to the resonance pattern of the patient.

The diagnosis is of particular importance in bioresonance therapy

And in bioresonance therapy this is possible because it works with the patient's own oscillations. A more precise treatment is not available. Even this precision

Exact treatment with the patient's own oscillations

can be enhanced because bioresonance therapy can lessen, or even delete, the oscillations of corresponding substances by using their oscillations in an inverted way.

Important factors for the bioresonance practitioner

The name of an illness from which the patient is suffering is not particularly important to the bioresonance practitioner. To him it is more important which functional circuits and organs are affected, whether allergic or inflammatory or degenerative processes are involved, whether the self-healing power of the patient is good or whether there are blocks in his self-regulation and whether there are only a few or multiple causes and triggering factors for the illness. To cut a long story short: the bioresonance practitioner in most cases has to establish an overall holistic picture of the health situation of his patient – even if he uses bioresonance therapy only as a supportive measure.

Which factors cause the illness or trigger it?

To do this he has to find out as many factors as possible that cause and trigger the illness of his patient and analyse them. First of all he uses the interview with his patient; after all in most cases they know their illness well and can give important indications. After that comes the physical examination that clarifies the symptoms. Extensive tests allow the real access to the illness. And finally results from laboratories and eventually a visit to the location – for instance in geopathic stress caused by a bed – round off the picture.

Holistic diagnosis

At the end of this process we do not simply have the name of an illness but we have gathered an abundance of information from which we can form for ourselves a holistic picture of the health situation of the patient. That is, the proper diagnosis which is the start of a (hopefully) successful treatment.

> The bioresonance tests are the centrepiece of this diagnosis.

Before we go into the methods of diagnosis in depth, you should know that they are completely different to those of conventional medicine, because their approach is on the energetic-informational level. For this reason they can lead to different, sometimes even opposite, conclusions.

Analysis of the faeces for candida fungus

As an example, I would like to mention the test for the presence of the candida fungus in the stool: a biochemical laboratory might under certain circumstances not find any candida because there is no candida present in the stool as such. At the same time, a bioresonance test might have a positive result because there is a candida oscillation present in the stool. However, in both cases there is a candida present in the intestines. (The negative result of the laboratory might be caused by the fact that at the time of taking the stool the fungus was only present in sacculations of the intestinal mucous membrane and thus not in the stool.)

Blood test for allergen-antibodies

Or: a serological antibody test (blood test) can have a positive IgE result, indicating an allergy. The bioresonance test has no positive result because the allergy information was eliminated and the substance that caused the creation of the IgE does not cause an allergic reaction anymore. Thus in this case the IgE test is positive although the allergy is not present anymore.

What is checked by the bioresonance tests?

The basic bioresonance tests

These are:

- The energetic overall situation of the patient
- The energetic situations of his/her acupuncture meridians (= of the body's functional circuit and organs)
- The influence on the patient of the oscillations of interfering factors of different types
- The effectiveness and tolerance of medication
- The optimal setting of the therapy device

The number of health-stressing, interfering factors in our industrialised nations is nearly unlimited. It is almost impossible to grasp them all. For this reason it is useful for a practitioner to follow a scheme for testing and treatment. Every practitioner has his own system. For my patients I hace divided the stress

Groups of stress factors

factors into the following groups:

1. Radiation
2. Toxins
3. Allergens
4. Micro-organisms
5. Faulty diet and metabolic disorders
6. Intestinal disorders
7. Physical damage
8. The psycho-social situation
9. Bad living habits

Long-term stress to the body's immune system caused by these interfering factors is a major cause of chronic diseases. Because they cannot be diagnosed by conventional medicine, they often are not known or recognised as the cause of chronic illness. In these cases a causal treatment is not possible and the treatment is limited to fighting the symptoms of the illness. But treatment should not stop there. Therefore, I will give you information about the main interfering factors in the sections below. These might be of importance in your case, too.

Which stresses impair health?

Stress from radiation

Radiation is energy that is emitted by matter (= condensed energy). It can interact with the organism when pairs of ions are created. In doing so it can have a biologically positive or negative effect. It can cause biochemical reactions and alterations of the body's own regulatory systems. Faulty regulation can occur when the oscillation pattern of the regulatory systems are superseded by external radiation, as happens in allergic reactions.

Geopathic interference zones

In general we define geopathic interference zones ("earth rays") as electromagnetic waves and fields caused by water veins, or fissures and faults, in the ground that are harmful to people. They have been known about for centuries and the "old Chinese" even took them into account in building their houses. Nowadays, their existence is being doubted by science like so many things that have been handed down from the past.

The electromagnetic radiation of the geopathic interference zones can have negative as well as positive effects on living beings and people. These arise from the interaction between the geopathic radiation and the individual field of a person.

Negative and positive effects

The influence of geopathic interference zones is strongest from stressing places where one stays for a long time, for instance the bed or the workplace. An expert dowser can establish the exact location of the stressing place and suggest a corresponding change that would ease the stress. But even a lay person can get a valid preliminary assessment whether his bed is causing stress or not. The following general symptoms are indicative:

- Problems getting to sleep or sleeping through, insomnia, restless sleep, talking in sleep, night-mares, sudden cries while sleeping, grinding or chattering teeth during sleep
- Excessive need of sleep, the patient wakes up tired, as if beaten in the morning
- Cold feet or legs in bed, freezing in bed
- Restlessness in legs during night, cramps in calves during night
- Perspiration attacks during night
- Health disorders that only appear during the night or increase during the night
- Breathing problems (possibly asthma)
- Inflammations of veins

On top of that the following special symptoms appear with children:

- Bedwetting
- Rolling the head, banging the head into the pillow
- Rocking the upper part of the body in bed
- Getting out of the bed

How can geopathic stress be tested?

The effect of geopathic interference zones can be tested in bioresonance therapy, for instance with the BICOM spin tester (a device with which it is possible to establish the left or right spin of the blood) or with special test ampoules like silicea. With these tests it can be established whether the patient is stressed geopathically. Evenly increased values of the acupuncture points of hands and feet can also be an indication of a potential geopathic stress.

Treatment of geopathic stress

If the result of the test is positive, the stressing bed should be realigned. If this is not possible in the short term, bioresonance therapy can offer bridging help by providing a BICOM skincare oil that has been modulated with the corresponding oscillations. This oil is applied to certain skin areas in the morning. This reduces the foreign oscillations that have been taken on during the night. (BICOM skincare oil is a special oil containing minerals on which therapeutic oscillations can be modulated.)
Bioresonance therapy should also be used after the realignment of the bed because it can shorten the regeneration time and prevent crises that often occur after a realignment.

Technical electromagnetic interference fields

Electromagnetic processes determine our lives. They control and regulate all physical processes.

Electric and magnetic alternating fields

Technical electrical alternating fields are created when wires are live. Technical magnetic fields are created when an electric current is flowing.
Electromagnetic radiation foreign to the body can influence the body directly or indirectly because it can be stored in the water of the body. It can also be emitted from substances that have been incorporated into the body. In any case, it can influence the body's own regulatory systems as well as the cell functions and cell structures. In doing so, it can interfere with the natural rhythms of the organism by superseding the body's frequencies – in an extreme case, up to a collapse of the cell functions.
Prof. Adey – mentioned before – writes that even rather weak electromagnetic fields can influence bio-

molecular systems such as the human being. He remarks that this can interfere with foetal development, cell growth and regulation, brain functions and hormone production as well as the immune system.

Harmonious and disharmonious oscillations

With external electromagnetic oscillations that enter the body, we make a distinction between harmonious (health promoting) oscillations, for example the Schumann waves, and disharmonious ones (disturbing the health), for instance the frequencies of microwave ovens. Electromagnetic waves and fields from pylons are a part of that radiation generally included under the term electro-smog. Electro-smog is emitted by a great number of technical devices and instruments. As examples we can mention: audio and video recorders, computers, electric blankets, electric kitchen appliances, electric clocks (radio alarm clocks!), TV sets, television and radio stations, cellular phones, pylons, radar installations, electrical wires in houses and homes, transformers and waterbeds with electric engines.

Electro-smog

Sources of electromagnetic radiation

They all emit electromagnetic waves that can negatively influence the regulatory mechanisms of people. Unfortunately there are no figures available on how big the percentage of people that react negatively to them is. This is not helped by the fact that physical trials of their effects are usually performed on people who do not belong to the risk groups, namely young, mostly healthy, male students.

In particular, the vast increase in microwave smog over the last few years has imposed chronic stress on many people!

The human being is an aerial for electromagnetic radiation

The human body is an aerial for all this electromagnetic information from the environment. A test to discover which form of aerial would be the most effective showed that it would be an aerial in the form of a human body with outspread arms.

You can test it yourself: if you touch the aerial of a radio that does not receive well even though it has been tuned very precisely, with your hand, you will see that the reception improves with you being an extension to the aerial. So in electro-smog, not only are the strong current sources that can harm the body directly important but also, indeed especially, the very weak ones. After long-term exposure even these can interfere with the organism because the body is controlled by ultra-weak oscillations – as has been scientifically proven.

Symptoms of electromagnetic radiation

A multitude of symptoms are caused, of which I only want to mention a few here: defence weakness, allergies, general weakness, disturbances of appetite, breathing problems, blood pressure problems, irritability, heart rhythm disorders, irrational feelings of fear, lack of concentration, headaches, development of cancer, multiple sclerosis, nervousness, depression, sudden infant deaths, period disorders, sleeping disorders, disturbances of sight, numbness and weakness in the legs, changes in body temperature, meteorosensitivity.

Unfortunately these rather general symptoms do not give a direct indication as to their cause being radiation. They can be very similar to symptoms from other causes such as toxic stress, allergies, inflammations, physical over-exhaustion and psychological stress. If they appear as a consequence of radiation it is very hard to recognise without corresponding testing whether the cause of radiation is geopathic interference zones, electromagnetic disturbances or radioactive radiation.

Electro-sensitivity and electro-allergies

Every patient reacts to different frequencies in line with his ability to go into resonance. For that reason some people are susceptible to electric current and others are not. Extreme sensitivity can lead to "electro-allergies" in which the patient reacts with allergic symptoms to certain frequencies that are typical for him (according to Prof. Cyril W. Smith).

Some people even react allergically to drinking water

Some people even react allergically to drinking water if it contains the allergising frequency! On the other hand, a frequency intentionally modulated on to the water can have a therapeutic effect. In addition, long term stress by 50 Hz frequencies (mains system) and by power lines, just from permanent exposure, is damaging for anybody.

Electromagnetic stress from the 50 Hz mains system

The important fact for diagnosis and therapy is – as

we have already stressed in the discussion of the term "resonance" – that in general only those frequencies that go into resonance with the organism have an effect.

Even people who are not sensitive to electricity are exposed to permanent electromagnetic stress and thus to the risks that are a result of the long-term influence of electromagnetic radiation. If exposed over long periods of time they can "acquire" an electro-sensitivity and they then belong to the group of electro-sensitives or electro-allergic people.

Long-term radiation can lead to electro-sensitivity

The intensity of the influence of electric fields on people can be judged on the basis of the level of the "connection tension". This "connection" states how much current somebody – for example, lying in the bed – takes on from his environment, for instance from a radio alarm clock situated at the headboard of his bed. This can be measured with an earthed voltmeter to which the patient is connected with a hand electrode. The value on the scale indicates the "connecting tension", for instance in millivolts.

Measurement of connecting tension with a voltmeter

However, this value does not indicate what effect the connection has on somebody. To judge this, his constitution, any other stresses, his regulatory ability and so on, also have to be taken into account. But these values can give a general indication whether the intake of current in bed during the night is tolerable or whether it will probably lead to additional distress instead of the necessary overnight regeneration. The factual stress can be checked with, for example, the test ampoule phosphorus (phosphorus in a homeopathic potency). In the framework of a general basic treatment, part of this incorporated radiation will be reduced but special medication can even have a more far-reaching effect.

Microwaves

What is the effect of the oscillations of microwaves? Normally the oscillations in the cells are in a harmonious co-ordination. This has to be so to make sure that all regulatory processes can function in an orderly way. The cell oscillation can be affected, as regards frequency and amplitude, by external radiation in such a way that it changes, increases, decreases or is extinguished. Subsequently, faulty controls of functions and biological rhythms or even the death of the cell can occur. Also the communicating signals with other cells are distorted: the complete organism is affected.

Defenceless against electro-smog?

In the highly-developed industrial countries the people are often defenceless against the influences of electrical and magnetic fields. They are powerless against pylons, railway mains systems and transformers. But in the home we can reduce the electro-stress by avoiding radio alarm clocks at the headboard of the bed, electric blankets, electric ring cables, metal bed parts, fluorescent tubes, night storage heaters and dimmers. Or at least banish them from the bedrooms.

Mains disconnector

With a so-called mains disconnector, you can interrupt the supply of current to your bedroom etc.. If installed correctly, the electromagnetic stress in bed is then nil.

Radioactive radiation

We have always been exposed to radioactive radiation, but until a few decades ago this was only radiation from natural sources such as cosmic radiation and earth radiation (terrestrial radiation).

The intensive effect of radioactive radiation

Only since the beginning of the technical use of nuclear energy has artificial radioactive radiation from military, technical and medical use, been added. This can destroy chemical compounds (molecules) and trigger an immense number of biochemical reactions in cells. One single particle of a beta ray can break up thousands of chemical linkages in the human tissue!

Every dose of radiation, no matter how small, can cause damage

If the radiation (for example X-rays) hits molecules in the cell plasma, numerous cell toxins can be created that can interfere with the cell functions or even lead to the necrotisation of the cell. Every dose of radiation, no matter how small, can cause damage. Frequent radiation with low dosages mainly causes long-term side-effects, once-off radiation with a high dosage causes acute damage. The probability of damage to the cells increases with the level of the dosage. In very high radiation doses, the destruction of the cell

membrane causes the cell to necrotise (this is the intention of radiation in cancer treatment).
It is impossible to estimate the overall stress of radioactive radiation. It is hardly possible to estimate correctly the yearly overall stress of natural and artificial radiation. It also depends on location, profession, way of life, medical care etc.

Measurement of radioactive radiation

The power of ionising radiation can be measured with certain measuring devices (Geiger counter, dosimeter, gamma spectrometer). It is also possible to measure with the bioresonance test procedure using a test ampoule (for instance, the test ampoule Aqua R 100) whether the patient is stressed by X-rays.

Stress from toxins

Toxins are poisonous or harmful substances that can make people ill. Natural substances, chemicals, medication, etc. are transformed (metabolised) in the body after they have been incorporated. The "clinkers" are excreted or stored in the body. In most cases the products of degradation are less toxic than the original substances, but it is possible for more poisonous products to develop.

Toxicity of substances

The toxicity of a substance for an organism depends on the concentration of the toxic substance, on the amount taken, on the location of its effect in the body, on the frequency and duration of the intake, on its division in the body and on the individual defences.
Patients who are treated with bioresonance therapy are nearly always suffering from creeping-chronic toxification that in combination with other stress factors has led to a chronic illness.

Summation and accumulation effects

In particular the summation and accumulation effects are important in the judgement of toxic effects. The single dose might be very small but the frequent intake of small amounts, for example from foodstuffs, leads to a summation and accumulation effect. This can be a real threat to the body.

The defence ability of those concerned is important

Of particular importance is the individual defence ability of those concerned. Somebody with a good con-

Risk groups

stitution is better able to detoxify and excrete toxins or, in an emergency to store them in the basic system without too many complications, than somebody with a weak constitution. This is why infants and small children with a weak defence system as well as people who have been weakened by illness, older people who have collected many toxins in their bodies in the course of their life, and also pregnant women and unborn children, belong to the real risk group of creeping toxification.

Inherited toxins

Venereal disease, tuberculosis and other toxic stresses of the ancestors (parents, grandparents) can stress the descendants in the form of inherited information. Their importance for the illness of the patient can be tested in bioresonance treatment, for example, with the test ampoules luesinum and tuberculinum. If they test positive, they should be eliminated with bioresonance treatment to relieve the defence system.

The volatile nature of inherited toxins

In general these inherited toxins gain their importance only in combination with other stresses, in which case they are a serious stress.

Toxins of the work place and profession

If the practitioner knows the profession and/or the working place of the patient this can give him important indications on potential stress from toxins.

Risk groups

- painters/decorators: evaporation from solvents
- hair dressers: chemical hair care
- gardeners: herbicides, insecticides
- housewives: cleaning agents
- laboratory assistants: chemicals
- farmers: pesticides
- metal workers: metal dust
- cleaners: chemical cleaning agents
- traffic wardens: stress from lead
- dentists, dental assistants: amalgam evaporation

The number of possible toxins is immense; because

they cannot be tested one by one some of the suspicious ones have to be detected in the interview between practitioner and patient and then tested by the methods of bioresonance therapy, for instance using the test ampoules benzolum with petrol station attendants or terabinthina (turpentine) with painters.

The effects of toxins from the work place and professions

Toxins from the work place and professions can lead to acute and chronic toxification and also to allergic and pseudo-allergic reactions. In particular, permanent confrontation with small dosages of toxic substances forms a creeping, but strongly rearranging, stress of the defence system.

Chloridated carbohydroxins

These days, damage by chloridated carbohydroxins (CCH) is in second place in the list of occupational diseases. Within this group the PCBs (polychloridated biphenyls) count as the most severe, followed by PCP (pentachlorphenol), formaldehyde and chlorine. With corresponding test ampoules they and many other toxins can be tested in bioresonance therapy without having to go the costly and time-consuming route of a blood examination.

- PCBs (polychloridated biphenyls) have been used in transformers, high-voltage transformers, paints, varnishes, softening agents for plastics etc.. PCBs are released into the environment through waste incineration. The same process can also lead to the creation of dioxins and furans.

  PCBs in food

  The production of PCBs has been prohibited in Germany since 1983. Nevertheless, PCBs are the most important environmentally harmful substances at the moment because of their presence in foodstuffs. Very small concentrations are present in vegetables and the most affected foods are fish and meat, in particular game and animal fats, because of their place in the food chain. The daily intake is about 2 micrograms from animal fats and about 0.5 micrograms from vegetable foodstuffs. Because they are highly soluble in fat, they are not only stored in the fatty tissue but also in the heart, liver, spleen, stomach, lungs and kidneys as well as in the adrenal glands. Because of their placenta permeability, PCBs can stress foetuses.

Symptoms caused by PCBs

The effects of PCBs are chronically toxic. Symptoms in humans range from acne to connective tissue inflammation and heart rhythm disturbances. A possible connection between PCBs and allergies is being discussed; scientific indications have been established.

Treatment of PCB diseases

A potential stress from PCBs can be examined in bioresonance treatment with a corresponding test ampoule. If the result is positive, it is possible to decrease or eliminate the oscillations that are stored in the body.

- PCP (pentachlorophenol) is a disinfectant and fungus-killing powder. It is also used as a wood preserver. Contamination with dioxins and furans increase the toxicity of PCP.

Symptoms and treatment of PCP

PCP can be ingested with food and absorbed through the skin. It impedes the energy transfer in the body. After long-term exposure emaciation, permanent tiredness as well as liver and kidney damage can result. A potential stress can be tested and treated with bioresonance therapy with corresponding test ampoules.

- Formaldehyde is, amongst others, a basic material for synthetic resin and plastics and a bonding agent for press-board. It is a textile aid as well as a disinfectant and preservative. But it is also contained in creams, cosmetics, shampoo, sealed parquet and carpets. It can also be traced in exhaust fumes and cigarette smoke. Formaldehyde has a toxic effect and, as an inhalation and contact allergen, can trigger allergic reactions.

Symptoms from formaldehyde

Contact with formaldehyde can affect the lungs, the skin and the gastro-intestinal tract. Joint pains, disturbances of brain function, headaches, tiredness and muscular pains are among the symptoms. Formaldehyde is justifiably suspected to cause cancer.

The test ampoule, formaldehyde, gives information about possible toxification. If it proves positive, the stress can be drained.

- Chlorine is a basic material in the production of solvents and inorganic chemicals. Further, it is used to sterilise and process water. Chlorine and its waste products are cell toxins. A corresponding test ampoule is available.

Toxins in the home and garden

Toxins galore

The home contains a multiplicity of stress factors, from wood preservatives and impregnating agents (for instance, lindane) through paints and varnishes (for instance, benzol) to old water pipes (lead). In the wider sense, furniture fabrics (e.g. tetrachlorcarbon), cosmetics (e.g. mercury), cleaning agents (e.g. tensides), carpets (e.g. vinylchloride), plastic cutlery (e.g. PCBs) and so on, possibly also tobacco smoke (e.g. cadmium) belong to the house toxins.
In the garden, chemical helpers are sprayed in the style of industrialised agriculture: herbicides, insecticides and anything else that can keep "weeds" and "pests" away from flower beds and borders.
Home and garden: hot-beds of toxic and allergenic chemicals.

Test and treatment of toxic stress

These and further potential toxification from home and garden toxins can be established with the corresponding test ampoules and, if the result is positive, treated.

Metals

We can divide metals into heavy metals and light metals. In general the heavy metals are more dangerous for the organism, but the light metals should not be overlooked as a potential source of danger. However, not all heavy metals are toxic, for instance zinc, iron and copper are essential for survival while cadmium, lead, mercury and thallium are toxic.

Serious heavy metals

In the experience of some practitioners, mercury, lead and cadmium belong to the most serious metallic stressors. For the practitioner, it is not so important that certain threshold values are respected, but whether a substance is damaging the defence and regulation ability of the patient at that point in time. This can be established with corresponding test ampoules.

Symptoms of lead toxification

- *Lead* can be found everywhere due to global environmental pollution. On average, 77% of lead intake is through vegetables and foods of animal origin, 14% from drinking water and 9% from the air that we breathe. Liver and kidneys (= the detoxifying organs) of animals are particularly contaminated with lead. Symptoms of a chronic lead toxification are lack of appetite, pallid complexion, slate-grey "lead-seam" on the edge of the gums, developmental disorders of the brain (in foetuses, infants and toddlers), impotence, headaches, gastro-intestinal problems, tiredness, nervousness, sleeping disorders, weaknesses, nausea, tremor etc.

Effects of cadmium

- *Cadmium* is an extremely toxic heavy metal. It is taken in principally through food (fish, cattle, mushrooms). Further source: tobacco smoke. Cadmium is suspected to cause cancer. Cadmium damages the defence mechanism and the nervous system as well as the detoxifying organs, kidneys and liver, the adrenal glands and the thyroid.
- *Mercury*. According to a publication of the World Health Organisation from 1991, the biggest daily intake of mercury is from amalgam, followed by fish and seafood.

Symptoms from mercury

  Mercury symptoms include allergic diseases, chronically inflammatory diseases of the respiratory tract, ocular damage, bloody diarrhoea, depression, dermatitis, fertility disorders as well as hormone disturbances and hair loss, problems with the inner ear, black mercury seam on the teeth, irritability, tinnitus, nausea, loosening of teeth and tremor.

Light and heavy metals can be tested for their toxic and allergising effect in bioresonance treatment. The detoxification and drainage of molecular sediments can be supported with bioresonance therapy.

Pesticides

Atrazine, lindane and parathion are amongst the most effective herbicides. However, they do not only damage insects but they can damage people as well. The material, energetic and informational parts of these and other pesticides interfere severely with the body's regulatory mechanisms.

Pesticides are a stress on the body's regulatory mechanisms

- *Atrazine*, which has been prohibited in Germany since 1988, was mainly used in growing corn to hinder the growth of weeds. Because it was used generously, it can be found in the ground and drinking water nearly everywhere, often in quantities not permitted according to the laws governing the quality of drinking water.
- *Lindane* is the commercial name for the pesticide gamma-HCH (gamma-benzene hexachloride). It is used in agriculture and horticulture, in household goods and in wood preservation. It belongs to the chloridated carbohydrates and like these it accumulates in the fatty tissue of animals and people, and in breast milk.
- *Parathion* (E605) is a strongly poisonous insecticide that is degraded to paraoxon in nature and in living beings. The paraoxon is the real and more dangerous agent. It is taken in through the skin, the mucous membranes and the gastro-intestinal tract. Symptoms of toxification are anxiety, asthma-like breathing problems, bronchial secretion, spasms, lung oedema, vertigo, perspiration, sialism, ticks and death through paralysis of breathing.

Test ampoules for atrazine, lindane, parathion and other pesticides such as DDT are available; the naturopathic detoxification of the body can be supported successfully by means of bioresonance therapy.

Detoxification with bioresonance therapy

Medicines

Medicines can put an additional stress on the organism. Unfortunately the expression "no effects without side-effects" is often proven true. Antibiotics, corticoids and the "pill" can contribute to the disturbance of the intestinal flora and promote intestinal dysbiosis and intestinal mycosis. Psychoactive drugs can block the regulatory mechanisms. Penicillin can lead to allergic reactions.

Medication is hardly ever adjusted to the individual regulatory ability of the patient, but as we now know the effectiveness of therapeutic impulses depends on the personal resonance. If this is not taken into account, the medicine will not work precisely and the parts that have no therapeutic effect can stress the body.

Test and treatment of stress by medicines

Prescribed medicines should be tested by the practitioner for their effectiveness and tolerance. This is no problem in bioresonance therapy. It can also diagnose disturbing oscillations of medicines that are already present in the body and decrease or eliminate these by inverse oscillation.

Vaccinations

Vaccinations not only protect, they can also damage. They can lead to over-reaction and to long-term damage to the organism.

Acute over-reactions

In acute over-reactions drowsiness, temperature increase, local inflammations, apathy, diarrhoea, vaccine eczema, etc. can appear. Acute vaccine damage can easily be recognised. It is harder to recognise the chronic, creeping damage such as disruption of regulation, that has been set off by the vaccine. Because every inoculation changes the frequency spectrum of the patient, a temporary consequence at least should be taken into account. This can still be tested years later as an interference.

Vaccinations can cause chronic stress

It is especially unfavourable if the vaccine damage is coupled with therapeutically suppressed children's diseases.

An example: a child contracted the measles. His natural healing was prevented by therapeutic measures that blocked the defence mechanisms. When he was vaccinated against the whooping cough, he overreacted. Now the suppressed illness, as well as the vaccine damage, block the defence system. These blocks can be lifted with bioresonance therapy by inverse oscillation of the vaccine.

Stress from allergens

A severe challenge to human defence mechanisms

Nowadays the defence mechanisms of most people living in the industrialised countries are extremely stressed. This is the reason why the defence system wrongly identifies more and more – even some harmless – substances as being threatening and sets off severe defence reactions, the so-called allergic and pseudo-allergic reactions. These reactions and the method of their treatment are described extensively from page 64 onwards.

Stress from micro-organisms

Micro-organisms threaten the previously damaged body

One of the most serious disturbances to health is to be infested by micro-organisms. These creatures draw their means of life from the human "host". However, in treatment it is all too often forgotten that it is not just the micro-organisms that harm people but that there has to have been some previous damage for the micro-organisms to become threatening. Only the damaged environment allows viruses, bacteria and mould to spread in an endangering way. The micro-organisms in this case are only the trigger. This is true even for AIDS and HIV.

Viruses

Viruses are very small micro "organisms" that cannot survive on their own. They settle in the nucleus of cells. Subsequent cell divisions take place with changed genes and only in the interest of multiplying the virus. It should indeed worry us that, for instance, the contamination of the population with the Epstein-Barr virus and with viruses of the Herpes group has already reached the level of 60–80%.

The treatment of viruses poses one of the biggest problems in medicine, for instance in therapy-resistant viral strains such as Herpes, certain Coxsackie and Epstein-Barr viruses.

Treatment of viral illnesses

The naturopath Martin Keymer succeeded in activating inactive viruses with bioresonance treatment and corresponding test ampoules, making it is possible to treat them for the first time. Conversely, he also succeeded in developing a procedure to render active viruses inactive to make them harmless if they are too much for the patient to cope with. This might be necessary to improve the defence situation of the patient, after which they can be reactivated and treated. It is also important for patients that the test for viruses is simple and does not stress them.

Treatment of bacterial stress

The treatment of bacterial stress is not as complicated as the treatment of viruses. Apart from a general stabilisation of the organism, it requires giving the organism the inverted oscillation of exactly those tested bacteria that constitute the disturbance. A large number of test ampoules and nosodes are available for this.

The treatment of moulds will be described in a special chapter (see from page 98 onwards).

Stress from poor nutrition and metabolic disorders

Proteins, carbohydrates, fats, minerals, vitamins and enzymes have to be provided to the organism in sufficient quantities and in the right composition to guarantee the maintenance of the body and to enable the body to fulfil its functions.

Malfunctions from disturbances of the mineral balance

One of these functions is the body's own regulatory ability. Imbalances in the mineral balance can change the "resonance" of the body in such way that faulty regulations will occur. Deficiency symptoms of essential minerals due to inadequate food (quantities and trace elements) stress the body just as much as a surplus. The disturbed balance of the minerals and the associated upset electrolyte balance, mix up the metabolism. This can lead to far-reaching malfunctions.

Along with the electrolyte balance, the water balance, the acid-base balance and the energy balance all shift. The "resonance body" organism also oscillates differently if the mineral balance is shifted. The ultra-fine electric currents of the unbalanced electrolytes form a new, distorted pattern. The scope of this book precludes inclusion of advice about an optimal diet here. In matters of diet, the expression "each to his own" is very true. The diet should be selected and prepared individually. However, one overall statement can be made: your food should contain as few artificial food additives as possible, because in nearly every case these are distorting factors for the body. Unfortunately, notwithstanding the obligation to declare them in all foodstuffs that have been produced commercially, not all ingredients are declared (for instance, not in bread, cakes and pastries) so that consumers cannot avoid all damaging additives.

Help from bioresonance therapy

Using bioresonance therapy, many damaging food additives, as well as some metabolic disorders, can be uncovered. The oscillations of identified allergising additives can be eliminated or reduced. It is also possible to treat metabolic disorders with bioresonance therapy. Nutritional shortages identified by tests can, in the short term, be compensated for with orthomolecular medicine, but in the long term it will be necessary to change the diet.

Clean drinking water?

One of the stresses caused by food is that from drinking water. The presence of harmful substances in drinking water matters, as well as its oscillations. Technically it is relatively easy to release drinking water from most of its unwelcome harmful substances. The best procedures are reverse osmosis and steam distillation. But even after cleaning (with reverse osmosis) you can still find in the water the frequencies of the harmful substances it used to contain. These oscillations can be harmful to the health and they should be eliminated. Additionally, the water should be energetically charged because in most cases it has become lacking in energy as a result of travelling through water pipes.

Stress from disturbances of the intestines

To some degree, the intestines, like the skin, are developed from the external (ectodermal) germ layer. This common source indicates their connection: skin and mucous membranes are barrier and defence organs. The intestinal mucous membrane separates the external (the content of the intestines) from the internal (the organs and the interstitial tissue). Therefore, coarse (high molecular) substances and antigens such as allergens, pathogenic micro-organisms and toxins should be prevented from passing from the intestines into the blood.

Excretory organs

Like the intestines, skin, lungs and kidneys are important excretory organs. The connective tissue is a temporary (or final) storage place for clinkers and toxins.

It is interesting to see that in classical Chinese medicine an energetic connection is postulated between four of them: large intestine (colon), skin, lung and connective tissue belong to the element "metal" and thus are element partners that mutually influence each other. This is the reason why in (electro-) acupuncture, as in bioresonance, by energetically influencing one of them it is possible to influence the others as well – a fact that once more shows us that the human being is one, holistic entity.

Lymph vessels of the intestinal wall

The intestines are the most important immunity organ of the human being

The intestines are the most important immunity organ of the human being. 70% of the body's defences are connected to the intestinal wall – the immune system of the intestinal wall thus surpasses the sum of all other lymphatic organs. Poor diet, antibiotic and cortisone treatment, intestinal dysbacteria and intestinal mycosis impede the reproduction and growth of the intestinal bacteria through a change of the environment in the intestines. Allergic or intolerance reactions inflame the intestinal wall. These factors, either on their own or in combination, decrease the immune activity of the lymph vessels of the intestinal wall.

Disturbed detoxification function of the intestines

The ability of the organism to excrete toxins via the intestines is connected to the functional ability of these lymph vessels of the intestines. If they are disturbed, so is the detoxification and excretion of toxins. The tailback of toxins in the intestines hinders the lymph vessels, and can cause a complete blockage.
As long as the lymph vessels of the intestines stay blocked, the intestines, and consequently the intestinal dysbacteria and intestinal mycosis, are resistant to treatment. Even a rehabilitation of the intestines cannot succeed in that situation. Therefore it is essential to restore the functional ability of the lymph vessels of the intestinal wall. In this, bioresonance treatment can offer a decisive contribution. Damage to the lymph vessels of the intestinal wall can be established with corresponding test ampoules and be treated with nosodes.

Intestinal dysbacteria and intestinal mycosis

The gastro-intestinal tract of the foetus is completely free of germs until birth. During and after birth it is populated with micro-organisms through contact with the vaginal mucous membrane of the mother and by environmental contact. Decisive for the composition of the future intestinal flora is whether the infant is breast- or bottle-fed. Each creates a different intestinal flora that largely stays that way for the rest of its life. Bottle-fed infants appear to be more susceptible to allergens because of their abnormal intestinal flora.

Causes of intestinal disturbances

The precarious balance of the intestinal bacteria can be further brought into disarray by a poor diet, medicinal treatment with antibiotics and other chemotherapeutics, as well as by infections with pathogenic micro-organisms. This then disturbs the digestion and the intake of elementary substances into the blood stream. As a consequence, an intestinal mycosis with all its far-reaching consequences can develop. Further information on this topic is contained in the sections on "intestinal mycosis" and "intestinal dysbacteria" (see pages 98 and following, and 106). Corresponding test ampoules are available for bioresonance treatment, for instance bacterium proteus, clostridium difficile, candida albicans, also aflatoxins of the mould aspergillus flavus interspersed through food that has gone mouldy etc.. In this case, the tested corresponding nosodes can also support the specific rehabilitation of the intestines.

Decay and fermentation

Decay and fermentation in the intestines are sources of high toxicity. They stress blood, liver and defence systems. The detoxifying organ, the liver, is flooded with toxins from protein decay, and alcohol from the fermentation hinders the degradation of other toxins, for instance environmental toxins. Without their elimination, no treatment can have a real, radical effect. In a lot of cases, therefore, it is necessary to test with the corresponding ampoules (for instance, bacterium proteus and alcohol). Reducing their pathogenic oscillations helps to relieve the organism.

Stress from damage to the body

Scar interference fields

Scars are like a dam in the connective tissue

Scars from injuries and operations with their cicatricial keloid (= scar adhesion) divide the nerves, bloodstream, lymph vessels and acupuncture meridians that run through this area. They are like a dam in the connective tissue.
Nerve impulses, bloodstreams, lymphatic streams and energy flows so to speak "go into blank space". This can lead to congestion and uncontrolled discharges at

the site of the scar. These in turn can lead to energetic disorders and pain. Because all functional circuits and all organs are connected to each other, an energetic disorder caused by scars can spread through the whole body, for instance in the form of rheumatism.

Suppressing interference from scars

With the test procedures of bioresonance treatment, it can be established whether scars form energetic interference fields. If so, they can be suppressed with bioresonance therapy.

Chronic inflammation as interference field

Chronic mandibular and sinus sepsis, chronic inflammation of the tonsils, chronic appendicitis, chronic joint inflammation, chronic abdominal inflammation and other chronic inflammations permanently challenge the body's defences. It constantly has to work to "hold down", to cope with, these focuses – and wears out more and more until it is exhausted. The endpoint of several long-lasting chronic inflammations is often a regulatory block or a regulatory paralysis. From here onwards it is only possible to influence the illness with great difficulty – if at all.
Because of the fact that an interference field has electromagnetic qualities, bioresonance treatment can check which chronic inflammations are active and whether they can be influenced therapeutically.

Dental materials

Dental materials can irritate the whole body

Amalgam, palladium and other metals – even gold – as dental materials can cause damage to the health. For this reason, testing for tolerance of existing dental materials is often necessary for the success of a treatment. However, before changing to new ones, the practitioner should check which materials the patient will tolerate.
In dental materials on a metal base the following mechanisms can lead to functional and organic damage:

Nature of damage

- *Abrasion of the material by chewing.*
Molecular metal parts can get into the stomach and the intestines with saliva and food. With the components of the food (for instance, proteins) they can pass the intestinal wall and get into the body via lymph and blood and from there into the connective tissue and organs. There they can cause toxic and electromagnetic cell dysfunctions. If, for example, they settle in the conducting system the effect can be neurotoxic disorders of the heart rhythm, or if they settle in the pineal gland the effect can be hormone regulatory disorders, for instance of the menstrual cycle.
- *Evaporations of metal due to oral temperature.*
The temperature in the mouth can cause metal ions to be set free and they too can get into the stomach and the intestine with saliva and food. They can also drift into the jaw through the oral mucous membrane.
- *Electrical potentials caused by different metals.*
Electrical potentials can develop between different metal alloys, such as amalgam and gold alloys, as well as between metal alloys and the oral mucous membrane. These electric currents have the effect of an electrolytic transport of metal molecules, for instance copper. These are taken up by the lymph and blood vessels of the oral mucous membrane and can either be stored there, or in the connecting tissue or in the organs.
- *Allergies caused by amalgam.*
Amalgam fillings can cause an electric over-sensitivity or electro-allergies. Damage to the defence system caused by amalgam can also lead to a general allergising. The symptoms of a creeping mercury toxification are many and mostly unspecific. They range from defence weakness through chronic migraine to a burning tongue. A complete list of symptoms would go beyond the scope of this book.
- *Brain scans* can be influenced by metal palate plates.

- *Further interference fields in the dental area* can be created by damaged teeth, paradontitis and paradontosis as well as dental granuloma. Dental fillings, damaged teeth and inflamed gums can have remote effects on the complete organism. If we see them as purely local problems we overlook this remote action. In particular the remote effects from the mandibular area can be a massive cause of chronic disease through the energetic connections of the teeth to the assigned organs.

Dentists who have been trained in the special dental bioresonance test programs can offer vital help. They can test the influence of acute and chronic inflammatory interference fields in the mandibular area, as well as of amalgam fillings and electric oral currents and other dental materials, on the health. Most of all, they can have a preventative effect by testing the probable effect on the patient of dental materials that might be used, such as gold, porcelain, ceramics and plastics.

Prophylactic tests

Maybe now, after you have read so much about interference fields and their potential consequences, you are asking yourself: how do bioresonance practitioners find out whether I am stressed by some of these interfering factors? To do this, several testing procedures that work on the energetic level are available to practitioners.

Bio-energetic test procedures

The most popular ones are:
- the electro-acupuncture diagnosis
- the kinesiology test
- the bioresonance test
- the Nogier reflex test

To complete the picture for patients who have already been tested with other energetic procedures, we can also mention that Decoder-Dermography, thermography, the energetic terminal points diagnosis, the segment electrogram and the VEGA-test can give valuable indications for bioresonance treatment. However, the results of the four test procedures listed above can be used directly in bioresonance treatment.

How do these tests function? What happens?

In a test, the practitioner tests what influence a substance has on his patient, i.e. he examines his reaction and his ability to react. The fascinating thing is that the body responds to every electromagnetic impulse. And this response can be measured. We will describe how this can be done.

Electro-acupuncture diagnosis

The electro-acupuncture diagnosis according to Dr. Voll (EAV) is based on traditional Chinese acupuncture. However, no needles are inserted but instead it measures the electric potentials of the skin in selected acupuncture points. In the EAV approach, as it is used in bioresonance treatment, these are mostly the beginning and end points of the acupuncture meridians situated at the tops of the fingers and toes.

Measuring points of bioresonance treatment

The reaction of a patient to certain substances is shown by the value of the indicator in the circular measurement scale at the front of the bioresonance device.

Testing disturbances

The values indicated give an insight into the extent of the disturbance of the measured acupuncture point.

A value that is too high (for instance, over 65 on the scale) indicates a high energy content of the measured meridian, which is the case in an acute inflammatory process (this can indicate a good ability to compensate). A value that is too low (for instance, below 50 on the scale) indicates a low energy content of the measured meridian, for example in a chronic degenerative process. If all the values are too high this might indicate an allergic occurrence or a geopathic stress. If all the values are too low this could mean that the body's self-healing power (the regulatory ability) is strongly reduced.

If in the test a stimulus is used and the reaction of the body to it is tested, then the practitioner can establish the patient's ability to react. He can establish whether the actual regulatory ability of the patient is good or insufficient. In testing medicine, the test value will go in the direction of the norm (towards the measurement value of 50) if the medicine is helping the patient.

A special test method is the "gridded test technique"

which, instead of testing the regulatory ability of the patient, tests his reaction to a therapeutic impulse. This method is based on the results of the research by the already mentioned Prof. Smith that therapeutic stimuli that go exactly into resonance with the patient have a therapeutic effect within a split second.

Kinesiology

Allergens, toxins, pesticides, medicines etc. can be tested by "kinesiology" on certain so-called indicator muscles. These are muscles in the body that can indicate how the patient reacts to certain substances, energies or even thoughts. In the kinesiology test, the patient can keep up the indicator muscle (for instance the right arm) against the pressure of the practitioner if the tested substance is acceptable for the patient; however, he cannot keep the arm up if the substance is damaging.

Bioresonance testing

In the bioresonance test, a tensor (a rod-like instrument with a movable top that reacts to electromagnetic oscillation) is used to establish the energetic relationship between two "information systems". These two "information systems" could be a patient and his potential allergen. (Please allow me to call a person – the patient – an "information system". In this test we are concerned with the oscillation = information that he emits.)

Two information systems could also be a food and a food additive if you want to check whether the additive is contained in the food. Or, if you suspect contamination with an intestinal mould, you can check the stool with a test ampoule containing the oscillation of the suspected mould.

In the bioresonance test the tensor will move up and down if the substance is damaging for the patient and will move horizontally if the substance is tolerated.

Nogier reflex test

The Nogier (or RAC) reflex test was developed by the French doctor, Nogier. It is a pulse test that indicates the reaction of the body (reflex) to substances that are being tested. The patient will hold the substance in his hand or he will get the oscillations via an electrode. The pulse is then tested for any changes caused by the substance.

The Nogier reflex test tests the "standing wave" of the blood. It is examined at the pulse point in the wrist. In the test, through the effect of the substance on the patient, the pulse wave moves for a short moment from the point where it is felt either in the direction of the hand or the elbow. This can be noticed as an increase or a decrease of the pulse wave. The practitioner gets his information about the effect of the test substance on the patient from this difference in the pulse wave.

BICOM spin tester

The BICOM spin tester is a special test instrument. Geopathic stress and substances (for example, foods or drinks) can be tested with it. The optical spin direction of the polarised light tells the practitioner whether they are advantageous or damaging for the patient.

Test ampoules

The bioresonance practitioner has a vast number of test materials available to him, which he will supplement according to the needs of his practice. The standard test ampoules for the diagnosis of allergens will be described in chapter 3 (see page 77).
Further test sets available are: bacteria, viruses, moulds, vaccinations, hereditary toxins, pharmatoxins, heavy metals, pesticides, environmental toxins as well as test ampoules for organs, meridians and "elements" from Chinese acupuncture.

The treatment

Bioresonance therapy: the energetic body treatment

Bioresonance practitioners know that body, mind and soul are one unit. They know that these are mutually dependant and influence each other in illnesses. Bioresonance therapy is an approach that affects the body. From there, through mutual effects, it also influences mind and soul.
The highest aim that a practitioner can reach is the restoration of the body's self-healing powers = ability to regulate itself. That is also the goal of bioresonance therapy:

> The goal of bioresonance therapy is the restoration of the body's self-regulatory ability.

To achieve this, the pathologic and pathogenic oscillations in the body have to be eliminated or reduced and the disturbed equilibrium of the cellular oscillations has to be restored. To do this the following effect has to be reached:

- Reduction of the disharmonious oscillation of the patient
- Reinforcement of the harmonious oscillations of the patient
- Reduction of the interfering factors that stress the patient
- Reduction of the oscillation of the interfering factors
- Reinforcement of the self-regulatory ability of the patient

The bioresonance therapy that is used to achieve this consists of one or more treatment steps per treat-ment session.

Basic treatments

Basic treatments improve the energetic situation

In a basic treatment the patient receives his own harmonious and/or his inverted disharmonious oscillations according to his tested energetic overall energy to improve his general situation and to reinforce his defence power. Thus also the regulatory behaviour of the patient is improved. Under certain circumstances a second basic treatment is added to give extra help to especially stressed organs.

Therapeutic impulses are always up-to-date

It is important to note the following: after the first therapeutic impulse, the oscillation image of the patient will have changed somewhat because pathologic and pathogenic oscillations will have been reduced. As the bioresonance device receives back these altered oscillations, it adjusts itself to the changed situation in split seconds. It adjusts the next therapeutic impulse to reflect the new oscillation situation. This adjustment happens again and again in the treatment until the disharmonious oscillations have been eliminated or

Patient and device form a regulative circle

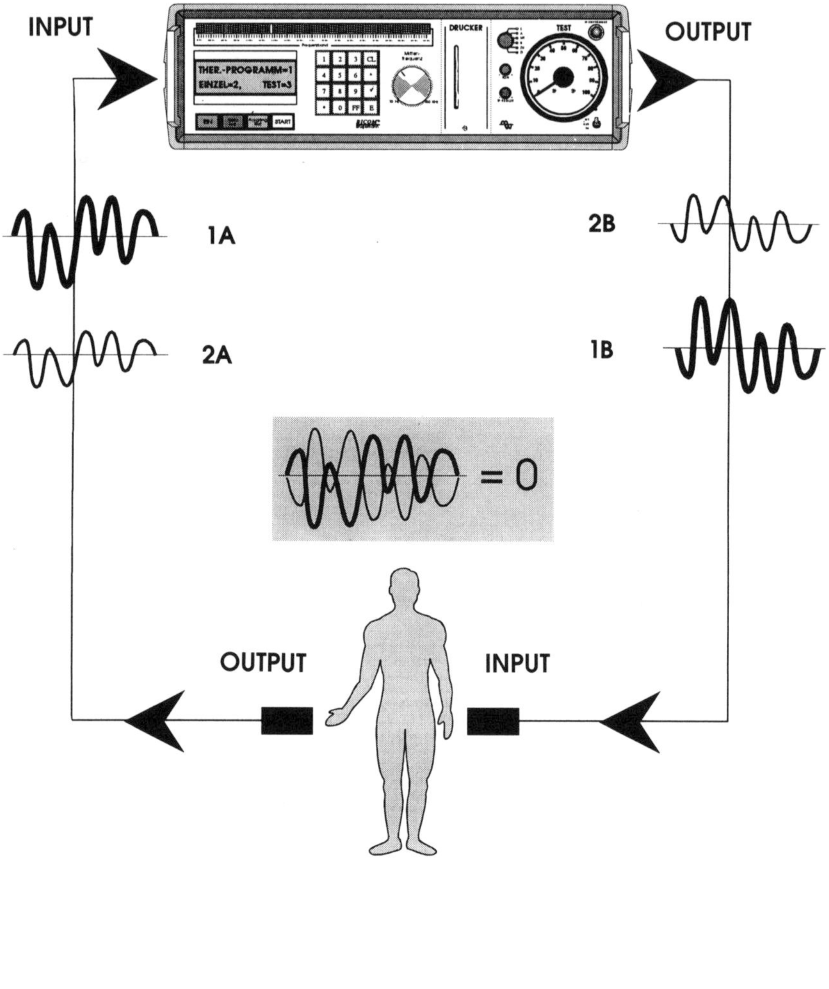

stress from disturbing factors has been correspondingly reduced. It is because of this ability to react that bioresonance offers a perfect individual treatment. The picture on page 56 shows the cybernetic control circuit that is formed. The strong disharmonious oscillation, 1A, that is fed into the device is fed back to the patient as a strong inverted disharmonious oscillation, 1B. As a consequence of the interference, the next disharmonious oscillation, 2A, that is fed to the device is already weaker and the returned inverted disharmonious oscillation, 2B, is correspondingly weaker.
Sometimes just one basic treatment without follow-up treatment suffices to stimulate the self-regulation to start the healing process. This is particularly the case with children who are only slightly stressed.

Follow-up treatment

Follow-up treatments are specific treatments of the stressing interfering factors

The basic treatments have an overall effect. The follow-up treatments are more specific. In these, the main stresses should be addressed and treated as precisely as possible. This can be done by treating the disturbed meridian or assessed functional and/or organ disorders. But it is also possible to treat according to indications (for instance, urinary tract infection).The oscillations of tested pathologic and harmonising substances are given to the patient. In the case of a urinary tract infection, for example, he will get the inverted oscillations of his own urine and additionally the oscillations of infection-inhibiting medicine via electrodes.

The body's own substances as therapeutics

The effect of basic and follow-up treatments can be enhanced by the use of the body's own secretions and excretions. These include saliva, sputum, urine, stool, perspiration (from head, armpits, body and feet), ear wax, nasal secretion, pus, a smear from the adenoid tonsil, skin smear, gastric juice, sperm, abdominal flow, tear fluid, vomit, the content of wound and burn blisters and herpes zoster (shingles) blisters. Blood also can be used for treatment.

Blood, secretions and excretions contain toxins etc. that can be used in the treatment by inverting the complete oscillations. Body fluids contain all the harmonious and disharmonious information of our body. They are ideal for a general stabilising treatment. Because their effect is often far-reaching, they should be used with circumspection so as not to overburden the body's ability to react.

In order to heal quicker and better after surgery, surgical matter such as extracted teeth, parts of bones, pathologic tissue, parts of the appendix, etc. can be used. The bottled substances are put in a brass beaker from where the oscillations of the substances are lead into the BICOM device via cables. In the device, the disharmonious oscillations are inverted and from there given to the patient as therapeutic impulses via cables and electrodes.

Individualising medicines

Medicines and injection ampoules can be individualised by modulating the patient's own oscillations on to them. These oscillations can be transferred through glass via thin cables and fed into the medicines or the ointment.

The therapeutic success of bioresonance therapy in infants, children and juveniles is very fast in most cases. However, adults are usually more heavily stres sed.

In chronic diseases especially, a large number of stresses are present. They often have to be removed layer by layer before the ability to self-regulate is regained. Again, in chronic cases the adrenal glands are often exhausted, and they have to be corrected first.

Individualising the treatment settings

Every patient has a personal oscillation spectrum. Consequently, he has to be treated individually. Most of the computer programs stored in the BICOM device are already individual because, in applying them in the treatment, the body's own oscillations are used. However, sometimes it is necessary to apply even more specific individual treatment settings. These can be tested on the patient using the following procedures:

- The question of whether the patient, in his given situation, should be treated with harmonious and/

or inverted disharmonious oscillations can be examined.

- Whether the treatment oscillations should be amplified or attenuated in comparison with the original oscillations can be checked.
- The length of the treatment time per treatment program can be checked.

The practitioner can adjust the treatment program of the BICOM device according to the tested values. The individual parameters are shown on the display of the device. If you are a bioresonance patient, you should have been able to observe this with your own practitioner.

Elimination or reduction of interfering factors

A precondition for a successful radical treatment is the elimination of stress on the body. Unfortunately this basic idea is all too often neglected. All interfering factors can put such great stress on the regulatory mechanisms of the organism that without their elimination, and/or without the elimination or reduction of their oscillations, a radical treatment is impossible.

Relieve regulatory mechanisms

Accompanying treatment

Many illnesses, in particular the acute ones, can often be treated successfully by bioresonance treatment alone. In other illnesses, combining it with other methods of treatment is useful.

Depending on the diagnosis and the goal of the treatment, these other approaches can be ones that work on the informational, the energetic or the material level. To list them all here would take too long and, in any case, every practitioner prefers different accompanying treatments in accordance with his overall therapeutic concept. However, to show you what is meant by "accompanying treatment", I would just like to mention phytotherapy, colonic irrigation therapy, dentistry and neural therapy. If you know which

Different concepts of treatment

accompanying treatment your practitioner uses, you can find out about it in one of the many books covering the field of natural medicine.

Successive treatment

After a course of bioresonance treatment is finished, it is sometimes useful to have a constitutional treatment. Normally this is done with homeopathic high potencies according to the rules of classical homeopathy.

Physical reactions to bioresonance therapy

Bioresonance therapy is painless and without side-effects

Possible reactions to bioresonance therapy

Bioresonance therapy is painless. To date, no harmful side-effects have been observed. Nevertheless, every now and then during or after the treatment reactions can occur of which the patient should be aware so that he can interpret them properly. The following varieties of reaction can develop: initial reactions, overflowing reactions, healing reactions, activation of chronic illnesses, and actualisation of earlier illnesses that have not completely healed.
This short summary is an overview of the different reactions:

- *Initial reactions.* The treatment of elderly people is much more difficult these days because of the number of toxins that accumulate in the body over a long period of years, for instance in the connective tissue. The growth of environmental pollution means we are increasingly observing high accumulations in young patients as well. This is why detoxification and the excretion of toxins have become important factors in treatment. If detoxification is not taken seriously by the practitioner and/or the patient and if not enough low mineral water is drunk (during the treatment at least 1½ litres daily) strong initial reactions can occur in the form of nausea, skin rashes etc. The more the patient and his excretion organs are stressed, the stronger and more disagreeable the initial reactions can be. So the excretion organs have to be activated! Detoxify, excrete! Drink a lot of water that is low in minerals, for example Volvic or (activated) reverse osmosis water.

- *Overflowing reactions* can occur if the patient is highly stressed, for example by geopathic stress. It can then sometimes happen that a treatment has a very intensive effect.
- *Healing reactions* usually affect the whole body. They express themselves in general symptoms such as a relaxed feeling, tiredness, sleepiness, warm feeling, but also cold feeling, moist skin, perspiration, fever, erythema, slight pains, inner uneasiness, and possibly speeding of the pulse or slight heart problems. These symptoms develop as a reaction of the body to treatment. They are a consequence of the physical "digestion" of the healing impulses.
- *Activation of chronic illnesses.* The healing of chronic illnesses usually occurs through their activation. To heal a chronic illness, the weakened defence system has to be reinforced in such way that it can actively fight the illness. In the process the chronic illness is "activated".
- *Actualisation of earlier illnesses that have not healed properly.* If an illness has been treated successfully by bioresonance therapy, a "new" illness sometimes follows. This is a nuisance for the patient because he thinks that the initial treatment was not successful, and for the practitioner it is often a riddle. In fact what is happening is that, because of successful healing, a better defence situation has been created and the defence system can now turn to an illness that has not healed properly before. This causes new healing reactions.

Report reactions!

The patient should report all reactions to the practitioner so that he can take them into account in the rest of the treatment.

Limitations of bioresonance therapy

Broad indication spectrum of bioresonance therapy

Nearly every illness is connected with disharmonious oscillations. This is why bioresonance therapy can be used advantageously in nearly every illness and there are practically no contra-indications. In most cases there is a chance of bringing about an improve-ment in even the most difficult diseases. So is bio-resonance treatment a universal treatment?
It is certainly a treatment with an unusually broad application spectrum, but, like other treatments, it has its limitations:

- Pathologic final stages, for instance the destruction of tissue, are impossible to regenerate, even with bioresonance therapy.
- Deprivation of minerals, vitamins, enzymes, etc. can impede the success of bioresonance therapy because in a situation of deprivation the "resonance human body" cannot go into resonance sufficiently.
- A patient who does not want to become healthy cannot be treated.
- Mental illness cannot be treated with bioresonance therapy.

Scientific proof

Understandably, the patient is mainly interested in whether he can become healthy with a certain treatment or not. In scientific medicine, however, it is customary to doubt even a successful treatment if it is not officially scientifically recognised. A good example of this is classic homeopathy that has been used beneficially for over 200 years. It still does not get scientific recognition because the people responsible for official recognition do not (or do not want to) understand it.

I mention this so that you know what it is worth if an "expert" tells you that bioresonance treatment cannot be worthwhile because it is not "scientifically recognised".

Is there, nevertheless, scientific proof of the effectiveness of bioresonance treatment?

Effective mechanisms scientifically explained

The first answer is the fact that biophysics is a relativly new scientific discipline that has not yet been acknowledged by conventional medicine. The way bioresonance treatment works can be explained in the framework of the findings of biophysics. Many high-calibre scientists like Prof. Addey, Prof. Popp and Prof. Smith produced experimental research results that help to explain the functioning principles of bioresonance treatment.

Proof from laboratory experiments

The second answer is the direct scientific proof of the effectiveness of bioresonance treatment. In-vitro experiments (in other words, experiments outside the body, in test-tubes) performed in the Oncology Institute of the Academy of Sciences in Kiev, Ukraine, resulted in unambiguous proof of the effectiveness of bioresonance treatment. Experts can request scientific studies from Regumed – Institute for Regulatory Medicine in D-82159 Gräfelfing.

Convincing results of treatment in everyday practice

A third answer is given by practice. A study performed by Peter Schumacher, M.D., of the treatment of 200 children suffering from allergies showed an 80% success rate for bioresonance therapy, which really is a considerable success for this illness.

Illnesses that can be treated with bioresonance therapy

Allergic illnesses

Allergies – the new illness of civilisation

Nowadays everybody uses the expression "allergy". A growing number of people react allergically to foods, pollen, goose down, cat's hair, fungus spores, ointments, insect bites, costume jewellery, cosmetics, cleaning agents or clothing.

The number of allergic illnesses has increased alarmingly over the last few years. They threaten to become an epidemic of civilisation. Statistics say that in Germany already more than 33% of the population suffers from allergic reactions. Illnesses such as

The spectrum of allergic illnesses

- nettle rash, chronic eczema, neurodermatitis,
- allergic sinusitis, allergic bronchial asthma,
- fluctuations in temperature, abnormal frequencies of the pulse,
- digestive problems such as flatulence, diarrhoea, constipation,
- allergic inflammations of stomach and intestines such as regional enteritis (Crohn's disease) and ulcerative colitis,
- allergic muscle and joint rheumatism and
- many psychological symptoms

torment more and more people. And in an increasing number of illnesses an allergic participation is being discussed.

The traditional methods are less and less effective

Unfortunately the chances of healing allergic illnesses drop as the environmental stresses increase. The traditional methods of treatment of allergies are able to ease the symptoms but they do not result in healing. The biochemically-oriented treatment of conventional medicine can make the symptoms of allergic illnesses disappear with chemotherapeutics (antihistamines, cortisones) and hyposensitisation (goal of treatment: decreased sensitivity to allergens by increasing the tolerance threshold), but it cannot really heal the allergies because chemotherapeutics and hyposensitisation do not remove the regulatory disturbance that is at the root of the allergies. The risk of further allergic reactions remains present.

The practitioners of the so-called clinical ecology can prevent the appearance of allergic reactions by allergy abstinence (avoidance of the allergens) and a rotation diet (each food is only allowed to be eaten once every four or five days), but they cannot remove the sensitivity to specific allergens. If re-exposed to the allergen, in most cases the allergic symptoms will reappear as long as the regulatory disturbance is not alleviated.

What can be done?

The traditional concepts of allergy treatment have to be scrutinised against the background of changed environmental conditions and the related increased stress of the body's own regulatory systems, as well as against the background of new insights into the factors causing and triggering allergies. In medicine, new diagnostic and therapeutic concepts have to be applied.

Allergies and pseudo-allergies

However, not everything that looks like an allergy actually is an allergy. In diagnosis and treatment a distinction has to be made between:

- an over-sensitivity, i.e. a stimulus response exceeding the normal level, for instance the development of cold sores on the lips from herpes after drinking from a glass previously used by strangers;

- an intolerance, i.e. a lack of defence against harmful substances, for instance a medicine, food or food additives, but also a lack of enzymes in foods that therefore cannot be digested;
- a toxification by harmful substances, for instance foods that have been contaminated with clostridium botulinum;
- a non-immunologic pseudo-allergy, i.e. a pathologic over-sensitivity that causes symptoms similar to an allergic reaction, for instance to a food additive;
- a real immunologic allergy, i.e. a pathologic over-sensitivity with an allergen-antibody reaction, for instance to cow's milk or grass pollen.

So what is an allergy?

You have probably already read a lot about allergies and maybe your practitioner has informed you about the current opinions, so I don't want to repeat things that you already know. I just will mention the basics and then concentrate on the new points that I want to cover in this book: the modern biophysical view of bioresonance allergy diagnosis and treatment.

Definitions from conventional medicine

Changed reaction

In 1906, the Austrian paediatrician Dr. Klemens von Pirquet defined allergy as "a changed reaction to a substance to which a previous sensitisation has taken place."

Faulty regulation of the body

Effectively, the body registers this substance as "an enemy" on the basis of a faulty regulation of the defence system and in subsequent contact responds with a over-reaction of the defence system. The consequence is a biochemical allergen-antibody reaction by the immune system.

Allergic over-reaction

The altered reaction of the organism can show itself either in over-reaction or in decreased reactions. These days an allergic reaction is generally understood to

be an over-sensitivity reaction with a propensity to over-react.
As you will read later, a continuing over-reaction leads in the long term to exhaustion of the defence systems and thus to an under-reaction. So it is also legitimate to consider an under-reaction as an allergic reaction, as was usual in the past. In the context of this book, however, I will always mean over-reactions when speaking of allergic reactions, unless I explicitly mention under-reactions.

Allergic under-reaction

The definition in biophysical medicine

In the last few years it has become clear that conventional medicine has reached its limits in the diagnosis and treatment of allergies. Allergies, as well as most chronic illnesses, are among the illnesses that cannot be satisfactorily treated by conventional medicine these days.

Allergies cannot be treated satisfactorily in conventional medicine

The reason for this is that the real causes of allergic reactions have not been studied in depth and the concepts of treatment have been too limited. In regard to allergic illnesses, as with chronic illnesses, conventional medicine is not able to overcome the "scientific" limits it has imposed upon itself.

What are the new fundamentals?

I would like to summarise:

- Allergic reactions are not only characterised by allergen-antibody reactions, but are often predisposed by a large number of stressing, interfering factors and finally triggered by one or more specific allergens.
- Although allergic reactions happen materially at the biochemical level, like all biological processes they are triggered and controlled by information at the biophysical level, in this case by the allergen information.

Antibodies

Degranulation

Mediator release

According to the findings of classical allergology, cells that have the potential to do so (certain lymphocytes) develop antibodies (immunoglobulins) at the first contact with an allergen. These settle on mastocytes. Following renewed contact with the allergen, a degranulation (fluidisation of granules in the cell plasma containing secretions) takes place through coupling of the allergen to the immunoglobulins settled on the mastocytes, as well as a mediator release (for instance, histamines). The vast number of mediators then causes the allergic reaction, as such, in skin and mucous membranes in the form of hives, inflammation, allergic rhinitis etc.

Allergen information

According to the findings of biophysical allergology, the allergic reaction is triggered by the information from the allergen. This decisive fact (which constitutes a big step forward in the diagnosis and treatment of allergies) was discovered by the Austrian paediatrician Dr. Peter Schumacher.

> The allergen information is pivotal in bioresonance allergy treatment. Only if you can influence the information, can you heal an allergy.

Contact with an allergen during abstinence can have severe repercussions

The problem is that an allergy information, once established, is retained so long as it (or its information) is not actively eliminated. This is clearly shown in the problem of the allergen abstinence: even if the patient abstains for months, a renewed contact with the allergen (for instance, hazel nuts) can re-trigger allergic reactions because the allergic disposition to this allergen remains despite the abstinence.

The stress researcher Dr. Hans Seyle discovered that a disstress (= a harmful stress), as an allergen is to the organism, initially triggers a severe reaction but that the organism can adapt to this disstress, as a continuing stress, for a long period until it is exhausted. He sub-divided the process into three stages that can also be used as a basis for allergic processes:

- First stage: the alarm stage

Immediate reaction

The organism reacts to contact with the allergen immediately or within a few hours. So an allergising food, for instance, in this phase can cause acute swelling of the mucous membranes.

- Second stage: the adaptation stage

Adaptation to the allergen

If permanently exposed to the allergen, the organism will adapt to the allergen and does not react obviously anymore. If an allergising food is eaten more than once in three days the organism adapts with a "chronic" defence to the allergen and allergy-specific symptoms no longer appear. The patient thinks he is no longer allergic to this food. This symptom-free adaptation stage is the dangerous so-called "masked" allergy phase.

- Third stage: the exhaustion stage

Exhaustion of the defence power by the allergen

If the consumption is continued the defence and adaptation ability of the organism becomes exhausted. Because of this exhaustion other interfering factors can have nearly limitless effects. Illnesses develop and nobody knows what is causing them so they become known as "illnesses of unknown origin".

Example

Let me demonstrate this whole process using the example of an allergy to cow's milk.

> After switching from breast milk to cow's milk an infant develops acute allergic symptoms such as vomiting and eczema. Because the mother does not recognise that the cow's milk is responsible, she keeps feeding the baby with it and with baby formulas containing protein from cow's milk. The child's body adapts its defence system to the permanent stress, the symptoms disappear and the mother is happy. (If she does recognise that the symptoms were caused by cow's milk she believes that her child now tolerates the milk. Far from it). After years of prolonged consumption of cow's milk protein, the child may develop symptoms in adult life that are caused by the exhaustion of the defence mechanisms due to the prolonged allergen consumption, for instance rheumatoid problems, migraine or depression.

Something similar can happen with any other food that is eaten often, whether it is a basic food like bread or "luxury foods" such as the "life-saving" cup of coffee in the morning, or favourite foods often eaten for pleasure such as chocolate, or even another allergen that the body is in permanent contact with such as dental amalgam.

The chronic allergies are in most cases "masked". For this reason, the direct connection between symptoms and allergens are often not obvious.

Masked food allergy can appear with any food

Masked food allergy can appear with any everyday food, with any favourite food and with so-called "luxury" foods that are eaten often. This means that masked allergy is the exact opposite of what is commonly understood to be an allergy: it shows no reaction or no reaction that can be attributed to an allergy.

Examples of masked allergies are neurodermatitis caused by allergies, bronchial asthma caused by allergies, inflammations of the intestines caused by allergies and rheumatism caused by allergies.

> "Masked" allergic illnesses are not recognised as such if the connection with the allergens is not understood. Therefore it is necessary to unmask masked allergies!!

Nearly every symptom can be caused by allergies

Allergic reactions can cause nearly all symptoms of illness

Allergic reactions can cause nearly all symptoms of illness and concern nearly all organ systems. To mention them all would go beyond the scope of this book. Nearly every symptom that brings a patient to you could also be caused by allergic reactions. For this reason, the practitioner should always consider the possibility of an allergic reaction in the treatment of his patients. I have described above how we can make a distinction between real allergies and pseudo-allergies. This distinction is important for diagnosis and treatment.

In a real allergy, the patient reacts to even the smallest

amount of his allergen. Under certain circumstances this can even be just the allergen information, for instance the steam from boiled milk.

Reactions to the smallest dose

In contrast to a real allergy, in a pseudo-allergy the patient reacts only after exposure to a larger quantity of a substance. The amount has to exceed an individual tolerance threshold. This is why the pseudo-allergy is a kind of "toxification" with the allergen.

Reaction to a larger amount of a substance

The following is to give you a clear overview of the starting point of bioresonance treatment:

Real allergies

1. Real allergies are triggered by even the smallest amount of an allergen, under certain circumstances even just the allergen information;
   - acute allergies are triggered by substances to which the patient is only exposed every now and then or only for a short period, for instance grass pollen, animal hair, aromas, strawberries, peaches, hazel nuts, medicines; ***Acute allergies***
   - chronic allergies are triggered by substances to which the patient is exposed daily or often, or with which the body is in constant contact, for instance foods such as cow's milk or wheat, goose down, moulds, intestinal fungi, mercury from amalgam fillings. ***Chronic allergies***
2. Pseudo-allergies are triggered by exceeding the individual tolerance threshold; however, they can also develop from a chronic, creeping toxification. ***Pseudo-allergies***

With food additives particularly, differentiation is sometimes difficult. They can create a real allergic reaction as well as develop toxic phenomena as a result of a summation effect, thus a pseudo-allergy.

Differentiation is sometimes difficult with food additives

As was previously mentioned, real chronic allergies are, for the most part, also masked allergies, the allergen character of which is often misjudged. Typical representatives of this category are neurodermatitis, allergic bronchial asthma and allergically-caused intestinal inflammations. I will discuss them below.

Neurodermatitis

The basis of the development of neurodermatitis is an

The disposition is the basis of allergic reactions

inherited disposition to react allergically. On this basis, a sensitisation is built up against an allergen which is in frequent – as a rule, daily – contact with the body. Dr. Peter Schumacher was able to prove that neurodermatitis is almost always a masked allergic reaction to a central allergen such as cow's milk and/or wheat. It is often accompanied by an infestation of the skin and the intestine with a mould and/or bacteria. The main foods, cow's milk and wheat, that are taken in daily from a young age are considered to be the most serious causes of neurodermatitic symptoms. Because of their central position in overall allergic occurrences, they are called central allergens and they probably form the foundation stone for many other allergies. This is why their treatment is of utmost importance.

Central allergens

Neurodermatitis caused by cow's milk protein

In our society, cow's milk is usually the first foreign protein that an infant is confronted with, be it direct or in the form of baby food that is produced from cow's milk.

The typical appearance of cow's milk neurodermatitis gives an indication for diagnosis for both practitioner and patient: as a rule, it starts directly after weaning or when supplementing with cow's milk while still breast feeding, thus in the first months of the baby's life. A sensitisation to mother's milk in breast-fed babies is also possible. Initially, eczematoid skin changes appear on the head and the face. These can be weeping and scabby. In later stages, these changes spread over the body, usually to the stomach and back, and to the extremities, appearing mainly on the anterior regions of the big joints. Weeping eczema is often infected with mould due to the scratching.

Symptoms of neurodermatitis

Wheat neurodermatitis

Wheat is generally the second foreign protein with which the baby is confronted (flour, semolina, rusks, as a component of baby food; later bread, cakes and biscuits, pastas). In particular, wholefood fans should consider that the continual consumption of wheat can lead to allergic reactions.

Symptoms of wheat neurodermatitis

Unlike cow's milk neurodermatitis, wheat neurodermatitis only starts around the second year, possibly even later. On the face, usually only the orbital area and the mouth area are affected, and the neck; on the extremities, mainly the posterior regions and the lower arms as well as the back of the hands. The eczema is mainly dry and often infected with mould due to the scratching. Wheat allergies are the most common cereal allergies. Allergies to rye etc. are less common. However, they also have to be considered in the diagnosis of neurodermatitis.

Candida neurodermatitis

The yeast mould, candida, can settle on neurodermatitic skin and aggravate the appearance of the neurodermatitis as an accompanying mycosis. (An accompanying mycosis is a mould infestation that is added to neurodermatitis.)

Don't overlook candida infestation of the skin!

If the treatment of the real cause of the neurodermatitis is successful, but the infestation with candida has not been treated, it will not be possible to ameliorate the appearance completely. It then may seem that the allergy treatment was not successful. However, in reality a residual mycosis that looks like neurodermatitis is still present. The one is an allergic component, the other the skin mould of the skin mycosis.

Allergies to candida mould

In addition, the body can react directly to intestinal mould in the form of an allergic reaction. In this case, the allergic skin symptoms have the appearance of neurodermatitis. It is, in fact, candida neurodermatitis. If it is not recognised as such, treatment will fail to address the cause and the neurodermatitis "cannot be cured".

Bronchial asthma

Chronic asthma, along with other respiratory diseases such as chronic sinusitis, chronic coughing and spastic bronchitis, can also be caused by allergies. The typical symptoms of asthma in this case have often already developed in children because of an inherited disposition to allergic reactions.

The diagnostic and therapeutic experience of bioresonance practitioners shows that allergic asthmatics develop two different forms of reaction:

Cause: inhalation allergens

1. "Superficial" allergic reactions
   As a rule the bronchial spasm is triggered by substances contained in the air (often in the form of suspended matter). Usually the symptoms are caused by inhalation allergens such as moulds, house dust, feathers (down), animal hair, grass pollen, dusts, solutions etc. used in professional situations, from children's toys (toy asthma), but also foods such as apples and nuts. Most asthmatics are multi-allergics.

Cause: ingestion allergens

2. "Central" allergic reactions
   Cow's milk and, in particular, wheat are the most common central allergens. These have to be especially considered if the asthmatic reaction appears after physical exercise, or is influenced by the weather, psychic stress etc. Reactions to superficial allergens can appear as well if these have superseded the central allergens.

The appearance of asthmatic illness depends on the measure of over-sensitivity of the patient, and on his overall well-being as well as on the effective power of the allergen and the intensity of the contact with the allergen. Previous damage to the mucous membrane also plays a role.

Regional enteritis (Crohn's disease) and ulcerative colitis

Causes that are often overlooked

Crohn's disease and ulcerative colitis, along with other intestinal illnesses such as chronic diarrhoea, chronic constipation and non-specific intestinal inflammations, are also illnesses that can be brought on by food allergies: allergies to cow's milk (milk protein and lactose) and wheat (wheat protein; not gliadin or gluten – these cause sprue or celiac disease with a degeneration of the villi of the small intestine).

With Crohn's disease/ulcerative colitis, intestinal yeast fungus stress is often present, which makes the

situation even worse. It is essential that this is treated otherwise a positive result will only be temporary.
It is striking that in many patients with chronic inflammatory intestinal illness, a chronic mercury toxification from amalgam can be observed.

When the organism is performing to its limit

Hyperergic allergic reaction

A hyperergic allergic reaction is a particularly strong reaction to a great stress. It develops if the defence system is challenged to the limit by the stress and builds up huge amounts of energy to cope with it. Such stresses can be caused by the intensive effects of

- radiation (for instance, strong geopathic interference zones),
- toxification (for instance, by heavy metals, dioxin),
- dental fillings (for instance, amalgam),
- allergens (for instance, cow's milk),
- inflammations (for instance, chronic kidney inflammations),
- micro-organisms (for instance, viruses),
- blocks in the connective tissue (for instance, by toxins),
- psychological stress situations (for instance, a lasting high-grade stress).

A patient in a hyperergic reaction situation can overreact to even the smallest impulse – unfortunately to therapeutic impulses as well as to pathologic ones. This latter creates a treatment block "on a high energy level" which can prevent effective treatment.

How to get past hyperergy

Of great help in overcoming hyperergy are the attenuation ampoules that have been developed for bioresonance treatment by the naturopath Martin Keymer. Using these, the high energy level can be brought down for the duration of the treatment.

Hyperergy as a healing reaction

Hyperergy appears with neurodermatitis patients, for instance, if they have already suffered from the symptoms for a long time and the organism tries to overcome the illness by increasing the healing energy.

Because of their highly sensitive reaction situation, these patient can react to minute quantities of their allergen during the period of abstinence. Experience has shown that they even react to immaterial impulses, for example to the steam from boiling milk if abstaining from cow's milk. This can lead to a strong dermatitic skin reaction.

Hyperergics often need to maintain very strict abstinence

If it is necessary to maintain abstinence before or during the allergy treatment, these allergics not only have to remove anything that contains their allergen from their diet, but also from their home and their environment. Just the handling of the allergen, particularly heating or cooking, can release the allergen information and lead to severe allergic reactions. So someone allergic to wheat also has to avoid bakeries, cake shops and cafés. Even grocery stores have to be avoided.

Hypoergic or anergic reaction

Hyperergy can affect the whole human being or just a single organ, organ system or functional circuit. In long-standing hyperergy a change to a hypoergic reaction (weakness of defence) or anergic reaction (no defence at all) is pre-programed. A serious chronic disease can be the result.

Allergens are everywhere

The number of allergens these days has reached astronomical heights. We can react allergically to nearly everything; natural as well as artificial substances. The unpleasant fact about it is that those substances that we suspect from the start can have an allergising effect, such as the numerous environmental toxins, but also such, in themselves, harmless substances as foods, flower pollen, etc.

Groups of allergens

Allergens have different "ways of entry" into the body. Because they have completely different clinical pictures, medicine has grouped them as follows:

1. The inhalation allergens
2. The ingestion allergens
3. The infection allergens

4. The injection allergens
5. The contact allergens

Combinations of allergens

It is alarming that the effects of allergens are obviously increased by their combination with other substances. Thus the combination of pollen with soot particles appears to produce a higher allergen potency.

According to data from the paediatrician Dr. Peter Schumacher from Innsbruck, an increasing number of children are developing allergies (nearly always inhalation allergies) to toys. Of particular importance in these cases are the polyester fibres (almost always from Asian countries) of cuddly toys or of shiny, washable and combable dolls (Barbie dolls, Ponies, etc.). They often have a distinct, aggressive, allergenic potential.

Asthma from toys

The symptoms of children who react allergically to these fibres are irritation of the mucous membranes with a permanently runny nose, inflammation of the connective tissue, and stubborn coughs. The occasional serious asthma caused by a reaction to toys has already been given a name: Toy Asthma.

If such symptoms occur in children, the parents and the practitioner should always consider the possibility that inhalation allergies and contact allergies have been triggered by toys. A short test with bioresonance treatment can give the answer.

Multiple allergies

So the spectrum of potential allergens is very wide. It is nearly impossible to give an estimate because once the regulatory mechanisms have been disturbed nearly every substance can trigger allergic reactions. Multiple allergies – allergies to more than one allergen – can be increasingly observed. Some people react allergically to over 40 different substances! However, these are often based on just a few central, main allergies. In that case, they don't necessarily all have to be treated; often there is no further reaction to any of them after a few of the main allergens have been treated.

Test ampoules

There are several test sets with test ampoules of allergens available to the bioresonance practitioner, for instance for pollen, foods (cereals, fish, meat, eggs, vegetables, fruits, nuts), insects, animal skins and mites. The practitioner will collect further test ampoules according to the requirements of his practice.

What are the causes of allergic reactions?

Currently, the development seems to go two ways:

Juvenile allergics

- On the one hand, the juvenile allergics whose physical and psychological stresses are still so small that the allergies are mainly triggered on the basis of their inherited disposition to react allergically;

Older allergics

The acquired disposition

- On the other hand, the older allergics who in the course of their lives have gathered so many stresses that the inherited disposition loses importance in comparison to the acquired disposition. With these people, multiple interfering factors both from their environment and internally, stress the body's self-regulatory mechanisms to such an extent that the organism can often no longer react normally.

Allergies are rarer in older people

It is an interesting fact that symptoms of allergies seldom appear in older people (let us say, over 60 years of age), because either the body has adapted to the allergens (the described phase of the adaptation to allergens) or the defence is somewhat exhausted and no longer able to produce allergic reactions (general defence weakness or exhaustion of the allergen defence).

> The cause of allergic reactions is, in most cases, a serious disorder of self-regulation caused by an overload of the body's defence. The allergens trigger the reactions.

However, in looking for the cause and triggering elements we have to consider not only the material factors but also the energetic and informational aspects.

Electromagnetic fields cause allergic reactions

From the point of view of bioresonance treatment, disturbances of the body's self-regulation are caused or triggered by pathogenic electromagnetic fields or, to be more precise, of corresponding information.

Stress from radiation

Stress from radiation (by geopathic interference zones or technical electromagnetic interference fields) is one of the causes of acquired allergic dispositions that directly affects the regulatory systems. It can be diagnosed using the bioresonance allergy test. Prof. Cyril W. Smith discovered that people can react allergically to electromagnetic fields directly, in particular to the frequency of the household mains voltage (in the UK 50 Hz), because they are exposed to it so often. If this is the case, normally sensitive people can develop into electro-sensitive people and then into "electro-allergics".

Electro-sensitives and electro-allergics

Stress from toxins

Toxic (for the organism, poisonous) substances have an effect at the biochemical level and, as a result of their oscillations, at the biophysical level as well.
Inherited toxins, toxins from industry and the work place, house and garden poisons, (heavy) metals, pesticides, certain food additives, contaminated drinking water, non-tolerated medicines, the consequences of inoculations, chronic inflammations, etc. also stress the defences energetically. Even very small doses can damage the immune system if they affect the organism for long enough.

Even small doses damage the defences

Those toxins that accumulate in the body through frequent exposure are particularly dangerous. They lead to a creeping "poisoning" of the body with increasing allergising.

Stress from food and food additives

We can react allergically to unprocessed foods, such as hazel nuts, and also to chemical substances that are connected to food. Industrialised agriculture and industrialised processing and production of food, stress the foods so strongly with chemicals and other substances that are foreign to the body, that in many

allergics it is possible to determine residues with the bioresonance allergy test.
It may be that the stress of the individual food is unimportant from the point of view of the food chemistry, but what really counts is the summation – or cumulative effect – of all foods that are consumed together. Two people who take in the same amount of a toxin can react completely differently to it on the basis of their constitution and their other stresses.

Increasing allergisation by food additives

Food additives are a creeping form of allergisation and poisoning of the organism. You can find them in cola-drinks, breads, cakes and pastries, sausages, canned fish, canned meats, any other kind of canned food, jams, fizzy drinks, sauces, soups and sweets. To cut a long story short: every supermarket is a minefield of allergens and toxins.

Stress from micro-organisms

Allergising by viruses, bacteria and moulds

Stress to the regulatory systems caused by micro-organisms is playing an increasing role in the development of allergic reactions. These micro-organisms are moulds, viruses and bacteria. By molecular changes to the DNA and by their oscillations, viruses can cause very severe disturbance of the cellular defences, and the metabolic poisons of bacteria do the same. Dr. Richard Mackarness was right when he proclaimed in 1975 that infections and allergies are directly linked. This mutual stress works in both directions.

Stress from disturbances of the intestines

Intestinal mycosis and intestinal dysbacteria

Intestinal mycosis (mould in the intestines) and intestinal dysbacteria (wrong bacteria in the intestines) are heavy stresses on the body's defences. All the evidence seems to indicate that intestinal mycosis, intestinal dysbacteria and allergies form one unit. How many allergologists take this into account?
A disturbed intestinal flora will be a contributory factor to allergies because of its electrolyte distur-

bance. Damage to the intestinal mucous membrane and the lymphatic vessels of the intestinal wall are also a major cause of allergic reactions because 70% of the body's defences are connected to the intestines. The intestinal mucous membrane, under attack from moulds, will be permeable to food particles and moulds that normally would not be allowed into the bloodstream. Once there, they cause allergic reactions.

Stress from damage to the body

Attacks on the skin and mucous membranes

Our external protective organ, the skin, is being threatened every day by shampoos, soaps, detergents, washing-up liquids, bath additives, etc., so that not much remains of its natural fatty protection. Foreign substances, for instance in cosmetics, can easily irritate it, or penetrate it, and thus lead to allergic reactions.

Our internal protective skins, the mucous membranes, are also constantly under attack. Tobacco smoke, suspended matter in the air (for instance, dust and lead particles), molecular soot particles, pollen, etc. constantly challenge the defence of the mucous membranes of the respiratory tract and contribute to their destruction.

The mucous membrane of the intestines is attacked by food additives, alcoholic drinks, medicines, etc.. Moulds settle on its surface and it gets infected. Molecular intestinal contents can enter the blood and the lymph system. Once there, they are allergens!

Chronic inflammations, interference fields from scars, etc., are stresses of the organism with a long-lasting effect that can contribute to irritation of the defences. Non-tolerated dental materials, such as amalgam fillings, are also causes or direct triggers of allergic reactions. I have already discussed this matter.

Clinkering of the connective tissue

The basic regulatory system – the soft connective tissue between the organ cells – is increasingly becoming the rubbish dump of the organism. Slags and harmful substances that can no longer be detoxi-fied and excreted by the over-stressed excretion organs –

intestines, liver and kidneys – are stored there. They interfere with the transport of oxygen and food to the organ cells; their oscillations disturb the regulatory processes and lead to allergising malfunctions.

Stress from the psycho-social situation

The psycho-social situation plays an important role in allergic illness

The psycho-social situation plays an important role in allergic illness. Maybe not the exclusive one as maintained by the psychosomatists, but it causes an instability. This means that the psyche is one among a great many stress factors and in individual cases may even be the decisive one as we can see in the development of cancer.

The suppression of the inner defences can lead to allergic symptoms

Thorwald Dethlefsen maintains that allergic symptoms are physical manifestations of suppressed inner defences and suppressed aggression. There are unpleasant events in an allergic's past which are not accepted by the conscious mind but which have an effect at a sub-conscious level. A remedy is the acceptance of the unwanted, in other words, the road of love. In my experience, allergies are even sometimes used to manipulate people.

Summary of the causes and triggers of allergic reactions

To end this chapter I will give a summary of the causes and triggers of allergic reactions:

- an inherited or acquired disposition forms the basis of an allergic reaction.
- the acquired disposition develops through an overload of the regulatory mechanisms because of multiple stress factors.
- these lead to the regulatory mechanisms reacting chaotically.
- the faulty reaction is then triggered by substances that the organism considers to be "enemies".
- with the sensitisation to an allergen, an "engram" is created on the informational level. Renewed contact with the allergen will activate it and lead to allergic reactions.
- the probability of allergic reactions depends on the allergen potency and on the question of how central the allergen is for the organism.

- the triggering of allergic reactions, as such, is caused by the electromagnetic oscillation of the allergen.

How to recognise allergens?

Interview of the patient (history)

Many patients know their allergens (for instance grass pollen or dust mite) and can name them to their practitioner. However, because they do not usually know their "masked" allergens, the ones they name are, in most cases, only a part of their allergic reality.

Laboratory diagnosis

Biochemical allergen diagnosis can uncover a large proportion of the allergens by immunoglobulin evidence in the blood and by skin tests. False positive and negative (therefore wrong) results have to be taken for granted. Also, in food allergies, the possibilities of biochemical tests are rather limited.

Bioresonance allergen test

Bioresonance allergen tests work on the level of oscillation. In them, one information system (the suspected allergen) is confronted with another information system (the patient). Their interaction is tested.

Different procedures

This interaction is displayed in various ways depending on the test procedure: in the allergen test with electro-acupuncture the reaction of the patient to the allergen is shown by the value on the indicator of the measuring device; in kinesiologic tests it is shown by the weakness or strength of the chosen indicator muscle; in the allergen resonance test, by the movement of the bioresonance tensor; in the Nogier test, by the increase or decrease of the pulse.

All these methods are highly sensitive procedures to test the energetic informational interaction between patient and allergen. They indicate whether a substance has an allergising effect on the organism or not.

Faulty measurements are possible

However, it has to be admitted that here, as well as in the biochemical test procedures, mistakes can happen if not all factors used in the test procedure are "right". Nevertheless, as a rule the energetic test procedures are correct. (Unfortunately there is no 100% secure test procedure at the moment – neither in conventional nor in biophysical medicine.)

Bioresonance test results give direct indications for the treatment

Bioresonance test results give the practitioner a direct indication of the necessary treatment. At the end of the test he will know which interfering factors need to be eliminated and neutralised to relieve the regulatory systems of the organism.

> The exact assessment of the allergen is a precondition of a successful bioresonance treatment.

Selective tests with specific test sets

Extensive test sets are available to the bioresonance practitioner, such as environmental toxins, bacteria and heavy metals. Additionally, each will compile their own test sets according to the needs of their practice (city or rural area, local plants and animals, bog or forest area, plain or mountains, etc.) and their patients (children or adults, profession, hobbies). To do this, the practitioner fills test ampoules with allergens or their solutions for use in allergen tests.

How to heal allergies

Depending on the situation, the bioresonance practitioner can try to eliminate the allergy engram directly or start with a more or less extensive elimination of the long-term stress factors and their interfering oscillations. Sometimes it is useful to include the holistic "five elements" theory from Chinese acupuncture in the treatment. (It is not possible to go into depth about this particular extension to bioresonance treatment in this book.)

Complementary therapeutic methods

Some practitioners exclusively use bioresonance therapy for the treatment of allergies, others complement it with other approaches used in their practice, for instance neural therapy, chiropractic, colonic irrigation, Bach flower therapy or counselling.

Thanks to the broad approach of bioresonance treatment, and the fact that it can be combined very well with other procedures, every practitioner can work according to his own therapy concept. Before starting a treatment, the practitioner has to have made up his mind about the following alternative possibilities:

- Is he dealing with a "superficial" allergic reaction, for example an allergy exclusively to strawberries or hazel nuts or meadow-grass pollen?
- Is he dealing additionally with a "central" allergy, for instance to cow's milk protein or wheat protein?
- Is he dealing additionally with a strong stressor that causes an allergic reaction, for instance amalgam, a geopathic interference zone or a candida stress?

In the first case only the "superficial" allergy needs to be treated, in the second case the "central" allergy has to be included in the treatment and in the third case the stressing, interfering factor and its oscillation also has to be eliminated.

Aim of the treatment

The aim of the treatment is the elimination of the allergen engram. This is aiming high because it means that, after the treatment, renewed contact with the allergen will no longer produce an allergic reaction. But even if there are good reasons why complete elimination is not possible, a lot is gained if the allergen information is "eased". In this case allergic reactions after renewed contact with the allergen will be reduced compared to the situation before the treatment.
The potential depends on four factors:

1. allergen power
2. allergen abstinence
3. the allergen information
4. the interfering factors.

Allergen power

Different possibilities to treat allergens

Some allergens are more powerful (effective) than others. There are allergens that mainly cause mild reactions, for instance, hazel nuts, and there are allergens that mainly cause severe reactions, for instance cow's milk protein. A powerful allergen is generally more difficult to eliminate than a weak one.

Allergen abstinence

In bioresonance treatment, there is "normal" abstinence vis-a-vis the allergising substance, and special allergen-code abstinence.

Normal allergen abstinence

Normal allergen abstinence is complete abstinence from the allergen, for instance avoiding a certain food or a food family for a certain period of time.

Special allergen-code abstinence

Special allergen-code abstinence also includes energetic and informational abstinence. This means: the patient is not even allowed to be in touch with the information of the food (for instance, the steam of boiling milk).

Nowadays, bioresonance treatment with BICOM technology is so far developed that strict abstinence is only necessary in cases that are especially difficult, namely if the allergen is a particularly great stress for the body's own regulation. Nevertheless, it is a good idea to avoid contact with the allergen before and during the treatment to relieve the body's defence systems.

Rotation diet

After the treatment a moderate form of abstinence is often implemented: the rotation diet. In this diet all foods are only eaten once every five days. This variety is intended to avoid new allergies developing against other foods.

The allergen information

A precondition for the elimination of an allergen information can be its deactivation. This can be reached by abstinence.

Imagine it this way: through abstinence the power of the allergen information is gradually reduced. Finally the information is deactivated. Now the elimination of the information is possible. After this the patient can take the allergen again without reactions. However, if the abstinence is broken, the information is instantly reactivated. The result is that the patient has

Activating and deactivating the information

allergic reactions again after contact with the allergen. If abstinence is not restarted from scratch it is only possible to reach an information relief, in other words, after the treatment the allergic reaction will simply be less severe than before.

The interfering factors

Relief of interfering factors

As I have said before, the multitude of assailing interfering factors is one of the main reasons for the increase in allergic reactions. For this reason, relieving the patient from interfering factors (avoidance of the interfering factors and decrease or elimination of their oscillations that are stored in the body) is often a precondition for a successful allergy treatment.

Case studies

Concluding this chapter on allergic illness, I would like to present three case studies, one each about neurodermatitis, bronchial asthma and Crohn's disease so that you will be able to recognise the essentials of bioresonance allergy treatment at a glance:

Neurodermatitis

The small patient, five years of age, had suffered from a generalised neurodermatitis with severe itching and weeping eczemas on the face and legs since she was eight months old. Her hair would no longer grow and her general health was very poor. The allergen test showed a central allergy to cow's milk. The child was in a hyperergic situation.
Because of the hyperergic situation, the treatment started with abstinence from cow's milk and, at the same time, a relieving treatment. After just one month a real improvement was noticeable in the face, the itchiness had disappeared and her hair had started growing again. Two weeks later the little patient came for a check-up. Her overall situation had further im-

proved and the eczema had further decreased. She was developing better and it was as if she had undergone a change. After a total of two and a half months abstinence, the BICOM allergy elimination therapy was started with the inverted oscillation of cow's milk. This was concluded three weeks later.
At the control check-up – one month later again – all clinical signs were negative and all pathologic skin afflictions had faded away.
At a check-up four months later the child's skin was clear and soft. The mother reported: "my child can eat anything without problems, even dairy products".

Bronchial asthma

A six-year-old boy had suffered from extreme asthma symptoms with a dry cough and typical asthma problems since he was a year old. He was using an asthma spray three times a day, needed inhalers and antibiotics, in other words the complete assortment of asthma treatment in conventional medicine. Using the test, a wheat allergy was found to be the basic cause of the asthma problems. In addition, the boy was hyperergic with extremely severe reactions to wheat protein. The treatment was started with a thorough wheat abstinence lasting four weeks. After that the child was treated with one basic and one relieving treatment once every three weeks.
Following the first treatment he continued to abstain from wheat but after about four weeks experienced a relapse, probably caused by a dietary mistake. Approximately two months after the start of the treatment his condition was very good. He no longer experienced any problems, no coughing, no asthma and in particular he did not need to use medication any more. His appetite was fine.
Approximately three months after the beginning of the treatment the weekly allergy treatment was started again. Everything went well and the patient felt completely well. About four months after the restart of the treatment he was checked again. The result:

not allergic to wheat any more. The patient could now eat wheat again.
Two weeks after the test his mother phoned and confirmed that everything was okay and that the child could eat wheat without a problem.

Crohn's disease

According to the 23-year-old patient, he had suffered from neurodermatitis as a child but was no longer suffering when his history was taken. An enteroscopy showed a strongly inflamed intestine with ulcers throughout the large intestine. He suffered from watery diarrhoea with between five and seven evacuations a day.
The tests resulted in an assessment of a central cow's milk allergy and a pollen allergy. The patient was hyperergic (thus a strongly-reacting allergic).
The treatment started with cow's milk abstinence and simultaneously a bioresonance relieving therapy every eight to fourteen days. During the abstinence and the relief treatment, there was a slow but consistent improvement. One and a half months after the start of treatment the patient only had three stools a day. These were already formed.
About two and a half months after the start of treatment the patient received a further eight bioresonance allergy therapies with the BICOM device. The results were very satisfactory: four months after the beginning of treatment the stools were completely normally formed and the Crohn's disease indications were negative.

Bioresonance therapy in human medicine

Examples of illnesses that can be treated by bioresonance therapy

Nearly all illness is either accompanied, caused or triggered by disharmonious oscillations. For this reason nearly all illnesses can be treated by bioresonance therapy with a good prospect of success.
Bioresonance therapy has proven itself in functional disorders, allergies, inflammatory as well as chronic degenerative organ and joint diseases, weakness of the immune system, any kind of pain, neuralgia, pre- and post-surgical pain, disorders of the hormonal cycle, accompanying treatment of tumours, speeding up of wound healing, any kind of injury, microbial illness, toxin excretion of industrial and household poisons, mycosis treatment, illness from dental materials, elimination of scar interference and treatment accompanying birth.
The illnesses described in this chapter will therefore be only a part of the overall indication spectrum. If you want to know whether any other specific illness of interest to you or affecting you can be treated with bioresonance therapy just ask your practitioner. Here I would like to thank all the committed bioresonance practitioners who, in the final analysis, have also contributed to the success of this book by sharing their experiences of bioresonance treatment in working parties and in congresses, in particular their case studies.

Rheumatic illnesses

"What you cannot explain consider to be rheumatism!" This satirical little phrase indicates that the illnesses making up the rheumatic family are plentiful. Among them are a number of painful and function-limiting conditions of the skeleto-muscular system as well as accompanying symptoms in other organ systems (for instance vascular rheumatism, dermatosklerosis).

Joint and soft tissue rheumatism

To narrow things down, a distinction is made between rheumatism of the joints and of the soft tissue, and in these between the acute and the chronic form. Acute joint rheumatism is accompanied by severe pain and fever. In chronic joint rheumatism the tissue around the joint swells, and although the pain is not so severe it is continuous. The temperature of the body hardly fluctuates. In soft tissue rheumatism the muscles and the connective tissue are affected.
The causes of joint rheumatism have not yet been fully explained. Because medicine tries to make a linear cause-effect connection, and these are subject to the latest findings in rheumatology, one theory chases another.

What is rheumatism?

It is a fact that rheumatism is a multi-causal illness, in other words a number of causes lead to rheumatic complaints. We find toxins, allergens, chronically inflamed interference fields (so-called focal toxicoses) such as tonsillitis, sinusitis, inflammation of the kidneys, dental root inflammations, also metabolic and hormonal disorders, intestinal dysbacteria, side-effects of medicines, damage from inoculations, hereditary stresses, etc..

The causes should be tested

In bioresonance treatment these possible causes are tested and treated accordingly, and the sediment of clinkers around the joints is checked.

A case study:

The female patient, aged 57, had suffered from rheumatic complaints for about 40 years. These became more and more severe as she grew older. The pains were localised, mainly in the muscles and the tendons, but she also suffered from a stiff back and from pains in the shoulder/cervical vertebra area. The patient's knees were often swollen. She also suffered from chronic sinusitis with heavy expectoration. Her sight got gradually worse and often fluctuated a great deal. She also often had problems with her gallbladder. As a result of her many ailments, the patient could only perform her duties as a cleaning lady in an old folks home part-time. The electro-acupuncture test, according to Dr. Voll and described above, indicated a massive allergy to wheat and a candida mould infestation. Unfortunately the patient could not keep to a complete code abstinence, which was ideally required in this case, because although she did not eat any wheat products, because of her work she was often in touch with them.

Ten therapies were given, each three days apart. After that the test for wheat was negative and the mould treatment could be started. The areas affected by the candida mould were treated with inverted oscillations of the mould and with oscillations of mould medicines. Three to four weeks after the start of the allergy treatment the patient observed that she was starting to feel better. Her mobility had clearly improved and her joint effusions disappeared. During the mould treatment symptoms of old complaints that had not properly healed before became acute, but after this acute phase they disappeared for good.

Her rheumatic complaints had improved so much that she started to enjoy life again. Before the treatment the patient was always so exhausted that she did not feel like doing anything after her working hours, but now she even took up a second job.

Further locomotor illnesses that can be successfully treated with bioresonance treatment

Further locomotor illnesses that can be treated with bioresonance with a prospect of success are arthritis and arthrosis, injuries of the joints of the foot, sprained joints of the foot, ankle injuries and swellings, swellings of the knee joint, hip joint problems, ischalgia, lumbago, sprained muscles, slipped discs as well as bone fractures and injuries. Of course in some of these bioresonance is not used exclusively, or primarily, but just as an accompanying measure.

Illnesses of the skin

The skin is a multi-functional organ. It has to carry out a number of tasks that range from the protection of the inside against external influences through duties to balance the temperature to detoxification and purification. For this reason about 80% of skin diseases are not actually diseases of the skin but "internal" illnesses that project their symptoms on to the skin. Therefore an external treatment will only give temporary relief as the suppression of inflammation of the skin by cortisone shows.

Most skin diseases are not diseases of the skin

What is required is the treatment of the causes that have lead to the skin disease. In this case, bioresonance treatment can help by:

Help from bioresonance treatment

- testing out the interfering factors on which the illness is based, for instance hereditary illnesses, allergens, intestinal moulds, skin moulds, intestinal dysbacteria, bacteria, toxic stress, functional disorders of internal organs, non-tolerated cosmetics, psychological causes,
- eliminating the oscillations of interfering factors,
- decreasing the pathologic oscillations of the skin inflammation,
- increasing the overall defence force of the organism,
- accompanying treatment, such as toxin excretion and medicines, to rehabilitate the intestines, activate the lymphatic system and detoxifiy the liver, plus treatment to build up the skin.

"Skin diseases" that can be treated successfully with bioresonance treatment are, for example, abscesses, acne, eczema, herpes simplex, herpes zoster and neurodermatitis.

Skin diseases that can be treated successfully with bioresonance treatment

A case study:

The patient, born in 1941, had suffered for several years from changes in the facial skin causing inflamed areas the size of pound coins. She suffered a great deal over her appearance. She made repeated attempts to find a cure but without success. Treatments for allergic reactions and the removal of amalgam, with an accompanying excretion treatment, were applied

but the skin phenomena could not be made to disappear. Because there was a suspicion of intolerance to metals, her bridge-work was also removed, but still the treatment did not work.
X-rays of her teeth only showed a root-treated tooth without changes to the top of the root. The bioresonance practitioner, who is himself a dentist, tested the patient using electro-acupuncture and found a dead root-treated tooth. This was responsible for the disorder that had already affected the skin over the whole head.
The patient learned from the dentist who had treated her before that the tooth had been filled with a certain root-filling paste. The bioresonance practitioner acquired some for himself. He extracted the dead tooth and started the after-treatment. In this treatment the oscillations of the extracted tooth were modulated on to the patient. Additionally an allergy treatment was given with the extracted tooth and the root-filling paste. These two treatment steps were repeated twice in the following week.
After the first treatment the red, inflamed patches were already nearly gone. After the third treatment it was almost impossible to see them. The patient could hardly believe this. After two more treatments, a check-up six weeks later showed that the facial skin was completely healed. Needless to say, the patient was very happy.

Illnesses of the heart and the circulatory system

Causes of functional heart disorders

The heart functions are controlled autonomously by the nervous system. This control is susceptible to allergens, toxins, electromagnetic fields, etc., that is, to all factors that can influence the control and regulatory mechanisms of people.

A case study:

The patient, aged 66, suffered from an illness of the coronary artery with heart constriction (angina pectoris) and radiating pain in her left arm. She also suffered from a decelerated heartbeat of 40 beats per minute and exertion pains in the chest. After a basic program, especially tested BICOM-programs were used to improve the heart activity, to control heart rhythm disorders, to detoxify the liver and for the excretion of toxins. St. John's wort oil was individualised with the patient's own oscillations (modulated) to rub on to the heart region.
After three treatment the patient was cured.

Illnesses of the lungs

In the process of breathing, we constantly take in part of our environment and give back part of our internal world: the air we breath. It is no surprise that the lungs in particular are endangered by environmental pollution and micro-organisms. The harmful substances in the air not only cause reactions of the bronchia and bronchioles but also enter the blood through the membranes of the alveoli.

Pollution of the air causes lung diseases

A case study:

The patient, 18 months old, suffered from acute asthma following pneumonia. To get the attacks under control, she needed up to eight inhalations per day. She was going to be taken to a university hospital for conventional medical examination but because the parents of the child heard about the bioresonance practitioner before the examination, they visited her before the appointment at the hospital.
She tested the child and found allergies to rabbit hair, doves, cats and grasses. The child was also stressed by viruses, bacteria and moulds and with hereditary toxins (tuberculosis). The rabbit and the doves were

kept by the family, and the child was often in contact with a cat at her grandmother's. The allergy to grasses was caused by hay that the parents made themselves every year.
The allergy to rabbits was treated with the inverted oscillations of rabbit hair, the allergy to doves with the inverted oscillations of dove feathers and excretions, the allergy to cats with inverted cat hair oscillations. For these allergies the substances of the animals to which the child reacted were used. However, the grasses were treated with the tested test ampoules. Viruses, bacteria, moulds and the tuberculosis stress were also treated with the corresponding test ampoules.
The child had five sessions, each two weeks apart. At the time of writing, over six months after the treatment ended, the child has not had another single asthma attack. She is doing well and lives completely normally without any limitations, as if she never had any allergies.

Illnesses of the liver and gallbladder

The liver does not feel pain

The liver does not feel pain, though the liver capsule can cause a distension pain. For this reason far-reaching functional disorders of the liver (for instance, disorders of metabolic and detoxification processes) or organic liver illnesses (for instance, hepatic cirrhosis) are mostly discovered very late. An energetic diagnosis is advantageous as an early diagnosis of disorders and damage.

Bioresonance therapy is also successful in the treatment of liver and gallbladder disorders

Many illnesses of the liver and gallbladder can be treated successfully with bioresonance therapy, chronic hepatitis and gallbladder colics among others.

A case study:

The patient, aged 60, was suffering from acute pains in the gallbladder area and in the right costal arch. Treatment started with a colour treatment. Subsequently the BICOM-treatment was started with programs that had been tested and with individualised therapy drops. The pains disappeared after just one treatment and they stayed away. Additionally, the sleeping disorders that he had suffered from for years and that had never really responded to any naturopathic treatment also disappeared.

Illnesses of the stomach and intestines

Main causes of gastric illness

The two most common causes of gastric illnesses are diet and psyche. Too hot, too cold, too fatty, too "heavy" foods, insufficiently chewed and insufficiently mixed with saliva, stress the stomach. Also, numerous known and unknown food allergens irritate the gastric mucous membrane, directly under which lies the layer of connective tissue with its blood and lymph vessels and the nerve plexuses. Because these control the production of gastric juices, functional disorders of the stomach often start as a result of nervous stress. When this is the case, we speak of a "nervous" stomach. Addictive substances (coffee, alcohol, cigarettes) also irritate the gastric mucous membranes.

Good results with gastric diseases

Gastric diseases can be treated very well with bioresonance treatment. Intestinal illnesses are often connected with the diseases of civilisation, allergies and intestinal moulds (intestinal mycosis). Their causes and triggers can be identified and treated very well with bioresonance test methods. However, treatment of intestinal diseases is often difficult and time consuming. In particular the illnesses Crohn's disease and ulcerative colitis, that are considered to be incurable, are often caused by food allergies and can be treated correspondingly with bioresonance treatment.

"Incurable" intestinal inflammations can be treated with success

Other gastro-intestinal problems that can be treated with bioresonance therapy are fullness, flatulence, gastric pains, diarrhoea, constipation, inflammations and ulcerations of the gastric mucous membrane and the intestines, intestinal dysbacteria, intestinal mycosis, intestinal fistula and haemorrhoids.

A case study:

The patient, aged 52, suffered from the symptoms of Crohn's disease: flatulence, spastic intestinal pains, heavy diarrhoea and complete loss of performance. In addition, he often suffered from hay fever. He had suffered from these symptoms "as long as I can remember". He had been treated by conventional medicine "since the beginning of time", but nobody had really been able to help him. As a result, in the six months before the bioresonance treatment, he had refused any kind of treatment. He simply lost his faith that anything would work. Finally, because of a recommendation, he went to a bioresonance practitioner.

Apart from the known hay fever, he also tested positive for milk and wheat allergy. His wife always baked cornbread for him, which was immediately banned from his diet by the practitioner because he could not tolerate it. The practitioner also banned the other "healthy" home-made breads, from which the patient got flatulence and bad breath.

From the start he was treated with the BICOM device and a BICOM add-on device (BICOM MRT^2) once a week. The allergies, the disturbance of the intestinal flora, the gastro-intestinal ulcers and the stomach were all treated.

After 15 treatments the patient felt incomparably better. The symptoms of Crohn's disease disappeared and he could eat anything with no problems. By treating the milk and wheat allergy, the hay fever also disappeared and he got through the first pollen season, again with no problems.

Intestinal moulds (intestinal mycosis)

Mould diseases have spread like wildfire over the last few years. Nowadays, nearly one third of the German population is considered to suffer from mould infestations.

In medicine, a distinction is made between localised and systemic mould diseases.

An organ mould infestation is the most dangerous

A localised mould infestation only affects one certain tissue (for instance, skin or intestines), a systemic one is spread through the whole organism through the lymph and/or the blood and then attaches itself to certain organs (for instance, in joints, brains, lungs).

Routes of infection

However, the affected area disguises the actual spread of the mould. Thus a foot mould (athlete's foot) can affect the intestines through the contact of foot-hand-mouth, and an intestinal mould can affect the sexual organs through a smear infection.

Systemic mycoses are particularly dangerous because they can affect and destroy organs. According to one statistic, in Germany 7,000 people die from such mould diseases every year. The number of unreported cases is probably much higher. This shows that mould diseases should not be played down.

Mould disease should not be played down

Mycoses produce unspecific general symptoms and organ-related symptoms: the general symptoms range from a general exhaustion through allergic reaction and general immune weakness, to itchiness and disorders of performance; the organ-related symptoms refer to the different skin diseases, illness of the mouth-oesophagus-gastro-intestinal tract, joint disorders, respiratory tract and lung disease, liver/gall disease, genital illness, nervous system diseases. A more detailed account of all symptoms would go beyond the scope of this book.

Simultaneous increase of mycoses and allergies

Particularly striking is the simultaneous increase of mycoses and allergies. One suspects on the one hand that both illnesses could have a common cause, on the other hand it indicates that these illnesses mutually boost each other.

Causes of mould infestations

Common causes can be found, for instance, in the careless prescription and taking of medicines with a lot of side-effects and, in industrialised society, food rich in additives. The mutual boost is caused by the fact that both illnesses weaken the defence systems and in doing so make it possible for each other to spread.

Moulds need an organic source of carbohydrates

To live and spread, moulds need an organic source of carbohydrates. Because they cannot produce it themselves, they are dependant on food for their supply. This can be in the form, for example, of foods containing sugar. Ideal for moulds are glucose, dextrose, cane sugar, fructose and maltose. Other good breeding grounds are refined white sugar and brown sugar, honey, maple syrup, sugar-containing juices, all kinds of sweets, bonbons, chocolate, biscuits, cakes, jams, jellies, ice cream, etc.; in general, foods containing sugar, as well as foods that are prepared with mould cultures.

Medicines as a cause of intestinal mould illnesses

Of the medicines, immuno-suppressive drugs, antibiotics and ovulation inhibitors pave the way for mycoses.

Immuno-suppressives

- Immuno-suppressive drugs (medicines that suppress the defence reactions artificially such as corticoids and antihistamines) are designed to weaken the body's own defences to block severe reactions, for instance in allergic, rheumatic and auto-immune illnesses as well as in the case of organ transplants. However, the inflammation-inhibiting suppression of the defences (immuno-suppression) fosters the spread of moulds.

Antibiotics

- Antibiotics (medicines to fight infectious diseases, such as penicillin and tetracycline) fight bacteria but at the same time damage the vital bacterial colonisation of the mucous membranes (intestinal flora and intestinal mucous membranes). Thus the defence power is weakened in an indirect way (the "exercise" of the immune system by certain intestinal bacteria is lessened); the vacated ecological niche is immediately taken over by intestinal moulds and the food now available is eaten by them. This happens with broad-spectrum antibiotics in particular.

Ovulation inhibitors

- Ovulation inhibitors (medicines containing hormones to prevent ovulation, the birth-control "pill") create a good breeding ground for moulds because of the hormonal shift.

Further causes

Further possible causes of mycoses that I would like to mention are:

- hormonal changes during puberty and in the normal menstrual cycle as well as in menstrual disorders,
- other hormonal preparations, also thyroid medicines,
- sexual intercourse and pregnancy,
- faulty hygiene, by antibacterial soaps and perfumed toiletries among other things,
- dysbacteria (damaged mucous membrane flora),
- diabetes mellitus,
- allergies, for instance to foods,
- toxic stress, for instance from heavy metals,
- infections, for instance viral infections by herpes viruses,
- defence weakness, for instance from chronic inflammations (the more severe the defence weakness, the more dramatic the mycosis),
- deficiencies of certain vitamins such as vitamin A, E or C, minerals (trace elements such as selenium, germanium, molybdenum), amino acids, fatty acids,
- psychological stress.

Risk groups

Who can contract a mould illness? In principle anybody at any age. However, the most susceptible are infants and toddlers whose defence systems are not yet fully formed, and chronically ill and old people whose defences are weakened. In elderly people, the bed-ridden are particularly at risk.

Mould illnesses are contagious

Mould illnesses are contagious, they can spread between husband and wife and partners and within the family. Possibilities of infection are, for instance, manual and oral contact, sexual intercourse, underwear, smear infections, and also the use of public toilets.

Mould fungus

According to the latest findings, mould fungi (for instance, candida albicans) are always harmful to people. A positive test in the intestines, or on the mucous membranes, or the skin is always bad. They can often spread very quickly in the body, in the worst cases they can double every 20 minutes. Because they can break through the mucous membrane barrier, they can get into the organs via the bloodstream – an especially dangerous situation. Additionally, they weaken the immune system. Dying moulds flood the body with mould toxins, and mould enzymes attack the defence cells.

Close relationship between allergies and mould and yeast fungi

Mould fungi participate to a high degree in triggering allergic reactions. The latest figures say that in approximately 80% of all allergies, mould and yeast mould are involved. Only a few practitioners and patients know about the frequent candida neurodermatitis quoted.

With mould fungi it is mainly the spores that are the cause of illness. They trigger allergic reactions of the skin (eczema) and the respiratory tract (asthma, allergic rhinitis). A complicating factor is that they can appear anywhere, not only in the house in carpets, wallpaper, wood panelling, old books, old materials, house plants, domestic animals (in particular birds), air moisturisers, air conditioning, but also outside. It is here, particularly, that it is becoming more and more obvious that mould fungi, apart from pollen and other air-borne allergens, are responsible for some inhalation allergies.

Among bioresonance practitioners, certain kinds of the yeast mould, candida, and the mould fungus, aspergillus, are considered to be the most dangerous for the body's own regulation.

The pathogens enter the body mainly with the air that we breath via the respiratory tract, and with food and saliva via the oral-gastro-intestinal tract. The defence of the mucous membranes is activated. The mucous membranes of the intestines have a special role: 70% of the body's defences are directly connected to the stimulation of the defence functions of the intestinal mucous membranes. Thus the intestines are not only an organ for the decomposition and intake of food but at the same time the biggest defence stimulation organ of the body. There are always bacteria on the mucous membranes of bronchia, intestines and vagina.

The intestines are the biggest defence organ of the human being

They are called bronchial, intestinal and vaginal flora. Apart from the mucinous film, they are a further protection against invaders and therefore are considered to be part of the body's defence.
If the communication of the body's defence is disrupted for whatever reason, then intestinal dysbacteria with all its problems develops. The treatment used to reverse the intestinal dysbiosis is called symbiosis control.

Symbiosis control

Treatment of intestinal mycosis with, as an example, candida albicans

Intestinal disorders with their distorted metabolic and defence functions are often a central cause of chronic diseases. The treatment of the intestines is therefore of particular importance. The following must be done:

Aim of intestinal mycosis treatment

- the destruction of the intestinal moulds,
- the reinstatement of the diseased intestinal environment (= symbiosis control),
- the curing of the damaged intestinal mucous membrane and
- the reactivation of the lymphatic vessels of the intestinal wall (the defence's place in the intestines).

In the treatment of the mycosis the primary aim is the elimination of the intestinal moulds. Without their complete removal there is a constant threat of a renewed spread of the mould, in particular if the mycosis diet is stopped after the treatment.

Complete destruction of the intestinal mould

At the moment the most effective method for the elimination of localised moulds seems to be taking Nystatin preparations and using the inverted mould oscillations. Nystatin inhibits the reproduction of moulds, for instance in candida albicans. In systemic moulds, systemic preparations have to be used.

Nystatin inhibits the reproduction of moulds

To support the fight against moulds it will be necessary in some cases to use so-called autonosodes of the mycosis. These are preparations that are produced from the intestinal moulds of the patient.
Parallel to the "destruction" of the moulds in the body and on the surface of the body by inhibiting their

reproduction, they are "starved" by a special mould diet. Normally this is based on the mould diet of Prof. Dr. Hans Rieth.

Avoid carbohydrates!

In the mould diet we are primarily concerned with the avoidance of carbohydrates such as sugar and all products containing sugar, potatoes, pastas, rice, etc.. Any products containing moulds also have to be avoided. Pork has to be avoided anyway because of its general lymph-toxic effect.

The mould diet has to be adhered to uncompromisingly, otherwise the inhibition of the reproduction by Nystatin would be quickly overrun by the high growth rate of the moulds. Deficiency symptoms have to be balanced and avoided by an individually adapted diet; under certain circumstances an acute lack has to be redressed by orthomolecular treatment (see glossary).

Repair the defence power!

Alongside the inhibition of the mould and the mould diet, the defence system has to be repaired. The reason for this is that the mould enzymes attack the defences in the form of mould toxins by destroying the defence bodies and thus rendering them ineffective. This destruction has to be answered by a specific repair, and the mould enzymes that destroy the immunity bodies have to be inhibited in their activity. At the same time the excretion and declinkering organs – liver, kidneys, lymph and blood – have to be supported.

Drink a lot of low mineral water!

It is particularly important to excrete the toxins and clinkers that have accumulated in the body by drinking 1 to 1½ litres a day of a still mineral water that is low in minerals (for instance, Volvic or reverse osmosis water).

Cleaning out the intestines is useful

Cleaning out the intestines (colonic irrigation) is useful because in this treatment the whole of the large intestine is flushed out, the faeces that contain moulds are removed and mould nests in the folds of the intestine are removed as well. Flatulent foods open up the intestinal folds and allow the water of the colonic irrigation treatment to reach into the depths. Approximately three weeks after the start of the antimycotic treatment the rehabilitation of the disturbed intestinal flora can be started. This is particularly necessary if an antibiotic treatment has been used prior to the development of the intestinal mycosis in which healthy intestinal bacteria have been killed as well as the pathogenic bacteria.

Rehabilitation of the intestinal flora

Patients who have had rehabilitation of the intestines already know that the leading bacteria, lactobacillus and bifidobacteria, are particularly important, as well as coli-bacteria. There are a number of preparations available for the recolonisation of the intestines.

The intestinal mucous membrane and the lymphatic vessels of the intestinal wall should be stabilised with regenerating organ preparations.

Mould enzymes damage antibodies

As has been said before, the mould enzymes (mycoenzymes) paralyse the body's defences. According to the experience gained up to now, bioresonance treatment changes the mould enzymes and their activity in such a way that they are no longer dangerous for the body's defences because they lose the ability to destroy the antibodies (immunoglobulins). For this reason the application of bioresonance therapy is vital in the treatment of moulds. Without inhibition of the mould enzymes treatment is often not successful.

Bioresonance therapy inactivates mould enzymes

In addition to the inhibition factor, the organism is reinforced defensively by bioresonance with the body's own oscillations. The application of the inverted oscillation of the tested moulds on the reflex zones of the stressed organs is another central and causal help in the treatment. The inverted mould oscillations can be modulated on to special mineral- and humin-containing BICOM drops and BICOM oils to be taken internally or rubbed on reflex zones.

Holistic mould treatment

Of course it is necessary to treat oral, skin and nails, and vaginal mycoses as well, to avoid relapse infections of the intestines.

Precaution

Finally it has to be said that the patient should in future avoid as far as possible the causes that led to the mycosis. By this I mean an uncritical use of immunosuppressives, antibiotics, and ovulation-inhibiting medication, and a careless diet. Instead of these there should be an increased use of naturopathic treatment and wholesome foods. More attention should also be paid to health-stressing environmental toxins and allergens. This is the best precaution against relapses.

A case study:

After three months of treatment with a dermatologist the patient, age 59 years, went to a bioresonance practitioner. Her hands, feet and legs up to her knees were covered with a thick layer of scales. Her skin was red and inflamed. The dermatologist had treated her with cortisone and had effected an apparent improvement. However, this only lasted a short while. As soon as the cortisone was stopped the old situation reoccurred. The specialist had not recognised that in this case the cause was a mycosis. For safety the bioresonance practitioner took a few scabs and sent them to the laboratory of Dr. Hauss. The result was as expected. It was a candida mycosis combined with an infection of trichophytum rubrum.
The first treatment the patient was given was an autohemo therapy, then a naturopathic remedy to rub in. Because of the seriousness of the case, bioresonance treatment was added. After 16 treatments the symptoms had completely disappeared. No relapses occurred. As a final remark: the practitioner advised the patient to destroy all her tights and to treat all her underwear and socks as well as those of her husband with a mould killer and to wash them afterwards. This was to prevent relapses through re-infections.

Intestinal dysbacteria

The micro-organisms of the intestinal tract influence the defence system and the metabolic performance in many ways. Some aerobic (depending on the presence of oxygen) and anaerobic (living without oxygen) germs such as proteus, clostridium, escherichia coli and staphylococcus can cause simple dysbiosis (thus faulty bacterial settlement of the intestines) or, in different combinations, mixed dysbioses.

Causes

But dysbiosis, as well as severe intestinal infections with intestinal inflammations and intestinal mycoses, can also be caused by immuno-suppressives, antibiotics, ovulation inhibitors, ionising radiation, environmental toxins, heavy metals and other toxic substances. A diet with denatured, industrially-processed foods, an unbalanced diet and food allergens contribute to dysbiosis. Psychological problems and chronic stress reinforce the interfering factors.

Symptoms

Flatulence, diaphragmatic eventration, heart problems, fullness, ulcerative colitis and intestinal cramps should make you think of dysbiosis.

Treatment

After a corresponding diagnosis, treatment is applied in several phases, this time without the BICOM device. In a pre-phase, preparations of dead symbiotic microorganisms are given, and in the first therapy phase, living lactobacillus and bifidobacteria. An autovaccination treatment (with homeopathised pathogen bacteria) decreases the number of pathogenic bacteria in the intestine. In the second therapy phase, preparations of living coli bacteria are applied, and possibly additional auto-vaccines.

Illnesses of kidneys and bladder

Tasks of the kidneys

The kidneys have to perform three vital tasks:

- They relieve the body of uric acid, urine, creatinine and other end products of the metabolism.
- They excrete toxins.
- They regulate the composition of the blood by maintaining the water and electrolyte balance and the acid-base balance.

Multiple causes

There are multiple causes for illnesses of the kidneys and the gallbladder. A multiplicity of causes can be held responsible for the different disorders from allergens, toxins and microbial infections to metabolic disorders. Bioresonance treatment is guided by the causal, stressing, interfering factors.

A case study:

The patient, aged 28, had chronic cystitis. At the age of 15, she had had an appendectomy and had suffered for many years from intermittent cystitis, increasingly so in the last two years. Despite allopathic medicines, she was in constant bladder pain.
The first treatment consisted of a basic treatment, followed by a program to re-balance a chronically degeneratively-disturbed bladder meridian and to suppress the interference of the appendectomy scar.
The second treatment also began with a basic treatment, again adapted to the energetic situation of the patient at that moment. This was followed by a second suppression of the interference of the scar and Bach flower remedy drops according to a test.
During the first scar interference suppression the patient experienced stabbing pain in the whole right side of her abdomen. After the second treatment she had no more problems with her bladder. A telephone call over a year later confirmed that she has not had any problems since.

Migraine

Severe headaches

The characteristic symptom of migraine is a spasmodic, severe headache. It is caused by cramping, followed by dilation, of the blood vessels of the brain. The folklore medicines (for instance, coffee) and medicines (for instance, ergotamines) might help in an acute attack, but are unable to heal the illness. This indicates that the reaction of the blood vessels is not the real cause of migraine but only a symptom of an illness on which it is based.
Could the other symptoms of migraine bring us closer to the discovery of these underlying causes ?
During an attack, many migraine sufferers experience stomach pains or suffer from vomiting, and certain foods such as coffee, alcohol, black tea and chocolate can trigger acute migraine attacks. Is the answer to

the riddle to be found in the foods? Could migraine be the consequence of a food allergy?
Clinical ecologists and bioresonance practitioners have studied this possibility extensively. The result of their research is: migraine can be caused by foods!

Migraine from foods

Often these allergens can be tested straight away with the allergen test ampoules. In the diagnosis of migraine the foods primarily concerned are those being eaten every day or very often, as you have read before. Occasionally, very rarely consumed foods are involved because these can also cause acute allergic reactions (the patient then is in the alarm stage). The foods that have been identified as being allergens can then be treated.
It also has to be taken into account which interfering factors have led to the allergic disposition of the patient. I have already discussed this topic.

Further causes

Further factors that cause and trigger migraine are: hormonal disorders; cervical spine trauma; inflammations, for instance of the gallbladder, the sinuses, etc.. These and other possible causes and triggers should be taken into account and tested and, if necessary, treated in the therapy for migraine.

1. Case study:

The patient, aged 45, had suffered from severe migraine with vomiting and vertigo, etc. for eight years. The allergy test showed an intolerance to cow's milk, cheese, tomatoes and coffee. First the central allergen, cow's milk protein, was treated, followed by a treatment of the stomach participation. After that, the other allergens such as coffee and cheese were eliminated.
Since the allergy treatment she no longer suffers from migraine attacks.

2. Case study:

The patient, aged 28, had suffered for a long time from migraine attacks that totally wore her out. In this particular case, the problem was unbearable. An examination showed that the patient had 17 amalgam fillings and a dead tooth. Over five sessions the amalgam was removed and replaced by a neutral cement. The dead tooth was extracted. (The practitioner is a dentist.) These rehabilitating measures were accompanied by bioresonance therapy and homeopathic remedies. After the removal of all the amalgam there was no reoccurrence of the migraine attacks.

Children's illnesses

Children's illnesses also have their good side

Even though they are a nuisance for children and parents – and dangerous as well if the fever gets very high – children's illnesses also have their good side. They exercise the body's defences and stimulate the formation of the defence systems. Use of antibiotics interrupts this process and, if repeated, can lead to a block of the defence systems. Further illnesses are then given free rein. For this reason in children's illnesses in particular, antibiotics should only be used in real emergencies and not as a routine prescription. In all honesty, there are enough other effective treatments that do not pose a risk. One of them is bioresonance treatment; the treatment of children's illnesses is one of its strengths.

Children's illnesses can be treated with bioresonance

The current topics of immunity weakness and susceptibility to infections play a big role in paediatrics. Young girls in particular are often in conventional treatment every few months with acute or chronic cystitis. The antibiotics that are often used indiscriminately block the formation of the body's defences and leave the children increasingly susceptible to infection.

However, using bioresonance therapy, the body's defences can be relieved and given time to develop. This means the body can cope by itself with subsequent illness. This way the child builds up its resistance, becomes sturdier and the constitution generally improves.

Broad field of indications

The spectrum of illnesses in which bioresonance treatment can be used in paediatrics is broad: acute and chronic, functional and organic illnesses and also illnesses that are only just emerging and could not yet be treated in any other way.
Bioresonance therapy can not only treat acute infections such as colds, sinusitis, middle ear infec-tions, throat inflammations, pneumonia, gastric illnesses, metabolic disorders, endogastritis, intestinal inflammations or pseudo-croup, but also their chronic forms and of course, most promisingly, allergies.

The hyperactive child

They are often a real pest for those around them and a riddle for their practitioners: hyperactive children. They fidget and jump from one chair to the next, clumsily knock things from the table, confuse the whole family with their machinations and disturb teachers and other pupils in school. They are insulted as being "abusive" and cheeky and they are considered to be mentally disturbed. But that is getting it wrong because their condition is pathological.
Hyperactive children have a pathologically excessive urge to move and simultaneously a psychological restlessness. They can display a large variety of symptoms and if we summarise these the developing symptom complex is called a syndrome.

Hyperkinetic syndrome

The symptom complex of hyperactive children is called hyperkinetic syndrome (HKS). It contains a bundle of symptoms that all concern excessive activity and psychological restlessness.

Fidgety as you like

Borrowing from the Keith-Conners scale, hyperactive children are characterised by the following symptoms, that do not all have to be present at the same time:
- They are uneasy, fidgety, impulsive, overactive;
- Their restlessness has no goal;
- They cannot sit still;
- They disturb other children;

- They do not finish what they start;
- They have sleeping disorders;
- Their writing is scribbley, chaotic, in extreme cases nearly unreadable;
- They move clumsily;
- It is easy to distract them, they are not focused;
- They want their wishes to be fulfilled immediately;
- They are easily frustrated;
- They cry a lot;
- Their moods swing quickly from one extreme to another;
- They tend to have tantrums and unpredictable behaviour;
- They develop cravings for chocolate, cakes, milk, lemonade, French fries etc.

Heredity

The development of HKS is probably based on a genetic predisposition (inherited). In genetically identical monovular twins both are nearly always hyperkinetic. In binovular twins, and siblings of a hyperkinetic child, there is still a 50% probability that these also have a hyperkinetic predisposition. If these predisposed children are affected by further severe interference factors the development of HKS becomes likely.

The main interfering factors that affect this development according to the naturopath Roland Schroeder are:

Organic brain damage

- Organic brain damage: during the pregnancy, and during and after birth, possible damage to the nervous system can promote hyperkinetic syndrome. A disorder in the phosphate metabolism in neuro-chemical brain damage could be an important cause of hyperkinetic syndrome.

Allergic stress

- Allergic stress: in nearly all hyperactive children allergic stress can be proven. These are primarily caused by food allergies and non-tolerated food additives. Top of the list are cow's milk protein, wheat, egg white, sugar, chocolate, candida mould and salicylic acid, but also phosphates, colourings, preservatives, emulsifiers, glutamates, sweeteners and fluoride.

- Toxic stress: inherited stress and toxins transferred from the mother during pregnancy appear to be the biggest complex of causes for hyperkinetic developmental disorders. In this, the pre-natal transfer of nicotine from smoking parents to the foetus appears to play a very central role, as do medicines taken by the mother during the pregnancy (for instance, tocolytics), and amalgam stress. Further toxic stress is caused by heavy metals, environmental toxins and pesticides. ***Toxic stress***
- Microbial stress: viruses and bacteria can cause severe stress that disrupts the sensitive regulatory systems. Directly illness-promoting are intestinal moulds (yeast and moulds) and faulty settlement of the intestines with pathogenic bacteria. ***Microbial stress***
- Geopathic stress: many hyperactive children are geopathically stressed. ***Geopathic and.......***
- Electromagnetic stress: this disrupts, among other things, the hormonal control centres in the brain. One effect of this is to cause metabolic disorders that can lead to disturbances in the intra- and extra-cellular mineral balance which increase the symptoms. ***....electromagnetic stress***
- Food: the number of allergic and hyperactive children has increased parallel to the change of diet to ready-to-serve meals and industrially prepared foods. A connection has to be suspected, particularly because of the increasing over-sensitivity to food additives in hyperactive children, as we have already mentioned in the chapter about allergic stress. ***Food***
- Deficiency in minerals: nearly all hyperactive children have a disorder in their mineral and vitamin balance. In particular there are often deficiencies in zinc, calcium, magnesium, sodium, potassium and vitamin B-complex. ***Deficiency in minerals***
- Metabolic disorders: a possible cause of the hyperkinetic syndrome is the over supply of phosphates through cola-drinks, chocolate, sausages, etc.. Often the cause is not an over supply, however, but a phosphate metabolism disorder. This in its turn can lead to a malfunction of the pancreas. ***Metabolic disorders***

Psychological stress

- Psychological stress: attempted abortions and the rejection of the child by the parents can increase the hyperkinetic syndrome.

An exact testing of the interfering factors is necessary for diagnosis and treatment because of the great number of possible causes.

Treatment with medication

In treating the hyperactive child, a therapy based exclusively on medication does not have the success that is needed and wished for, and the same goes for a purely diet-oriented or psychological treatment. Because of the large number of possible causes, a holistic approach is called for. The basis of this is an extensive history and careful tests. A treatment plan involving bioresonance therapy could include the following areas:

Holistic therapy plan

- treatment of allergic stress,
- treatment of toxic stress,
- treatment of microbial stress,
- treatment of geopathic stress,
- treatment of electromagnetic stress,
- treatment of intestinal mycosis,
- treatment of intestinal dysbacteria,
- treatment of metabolic disorders,
- balancing deficiencies of the diet,
- treatment of stressed organs,
- treatment of chronic interference fields,
- treatment of psychological stress.

As accompanying or follow-up treatment the following can be useful depending on the specific situation: physiotherapy, kinesiologic exercises, Bach flower therapy, constitutional therapy with homeopathic singular remedies, specific allergy diet, and homeopathic or phytotherapeutic remedies that support the excretion organs.

Feminine illnesses

Hormonally and neuro-vegetatively caused problems

Patients with hormonal and neuro-vegetative disorders visit the gynaecologist every day exhibiting, for example, menstrual problems or fertility disorders.

These patients report accompanying problems such as occasional headaches, heart problems, circulatory problems, gastro-intestinal problems, mood and weight swings, in other words symptoms that indicate an all-round regulatory disorder of the pineal and pituitary glands.

A case study:

A young woman patient suffered from menstrual cramps for years. She had a very small, under-developed womb. During her periods, she got severe cramps and always had to stay in bed for two days with a hot water bottle on her stomach. She was often nauseous as well. Neither homeopathy nor hormonal treatment were able to help her.
She came to the practice with acute menstruation problems. After the basic treatment, she was treated with a specific BICOM menstruation program that included the use of her menstrual flow. Immediately after the treatment the pains stopped. To make sure, she was treated again the following day.
The young woman reported that the problems were a lot less severe during her next period. She was treated again as described since when she has stayed almost completely free of problems.
For the treating gynaecologist this was not an isolated case. He reports that he can successfully help nearly all his patients who have similar problems using bioresonance treatment.

Tumour diseases

Bioresonance as an accompanying treatment in cancer treatment

If we accept that all illnesses are accompanied by disharmonious oscillations and that the reduction or elimination of these at the very least relieves the body's defence system, then bioresonance treatment should also be applicable in the treatment of cancer. Indeed this has proved to be the case in practices which treat cancer patients. This is why I want to report two out of a number of successful bioresonance cancer treatments. The success to date gives hope for a possible improvement of the usual cancer treatment.

1. Case study:

The gynaecologist, using ultrasound, had diagnosed a walnut-sized tumour in the right breast of a 34-year-old patient (breast cancer). He requested an immediate operation because the malignancy of the tumour was ascertained by a puncture biopsy. However, the patient insisted on a bioresonance treatment. The initial decoder picture made by the bioresonance practitioner showed inflammatory signs in the head-breast region.
The patient was treated three times per week. Initially, a tested basic program was applied for a month and subsequently a specific, supporting, cancer program. Additionally, at each treatment substances from her own body were used, such as saliva, blood, urine or faeces according to tests.
During the next six months she was treated with individual programs and tested body substances as well as with modulated cancer nosodes. Viral stress was treated with the BICOM-device and stabilising substances were modulated. Her candida infestation was also treated. A supplementary therapy with the MULTICOM device (see glossary) proved useful.
During the first week of treatment the patient got a severe, purulent acne on her face and chest which did not disappear until five months later.
Eight months after the start of her treatment she went back to her gynaecologist who could no longer find a tumour by ultrasound. However, the treatment with the bioresonance practitioner continued until the decoder picture also showed the all clear.

2. Case study:

The man, aged 34, had suffered for approximately six months from Hodgkin's lymphoma (a malignant

illness of the lymphatic system). He had been treated clinically with chemotherapy – he had lost his hair, and looked so grey and miserable that the bioresonance practitioner did not think at first she could do anything for him at all.
The practitioner approached the case very carefully. First, she defined the goals of her treatment:

- strengthen the immune system,
- influence the anaemia,
- create a new will to live.

In the treatment she used the special accompanying BICOM tumour program as well as the BICOM iron metabolism program, and several other programs for basic treatment. In addition, the patient received naturopathic medication. During the second and third treatments a therapy with the MULTICOM device and a reflexology massage were added.
After only the first week of therapy the patient had lost most of his grey, pale appearance. After the third session, he was released from bioresonance treatment and put into clinical therapy.
When he came to the practice for the next series of treatments, the practitioner could hardly believe her eyes: before her stood a young man with strong black hair – somebody who did not look ill at all. The values of the laboratory tests had almost normalised as well. A second series of treatments was now applied that strengthened the patient even more. The next treatment was planned for four months later. Shortly before that the patient called and said that he had been released from the clinic as being "healed".
This system of treatment has proved its value in many other cases, too.

The teeth

Dental and mandibular illness can block healing

In chronic illness, the oral and mandibular areas are often overlooked in diagnosis and treatment. However, healing often depends on these areas.
The energetic-informational relationship between teeth

and organs is known to most naturopathic-oriented practitioners. Dead teeth, ulcerations of the top of the dental root, mandibular inflammations and amalgam or palladium stress as well as other non-tolerated dental materials can stress the organs that are connected to the teeth so severely that without their rehabilitation a successful treatment is impossible.

Interaction between teeth and organs

It is possible to find these interfering factors with bioresonance treatment and to have them alleviated by a dentist who works biologically. Additionally, bioresonance therapy can speed up the healing of wounds after dental extractions and operations. Tolerance to materials to be used in any kind of dental treatment can be tested in advance.

A case study:

The patient complained about a cervical disc that kept slipping. She could not move her head sideways and she had the feeling that there was a clamp around her heart. The doctor could not find anything but a few extra systoles every now and then that were pathologically insignificant. So the patient was advised to seek psychiatric help, which she obviously refused.

Tests by a bioresonance practitioner showed a clear amalgam stress and a chronic inflammation of the sinuses. At the request of the patient the treatment was applied with as little medication as possible, so in the initial stage of the treatment the practitioner applied a neural therapy to ease the acute problems alongside the bioresonance therapy.

The patient was initially treated with a BICOM therapy program for chronic sinusitis, and a sinus nosode. Lymph remedies and kidney teas were also applied. After three months the patient could move her head again and no longer suffered from vertebral prolapses.

Then, after an initial bioresonance therapy, the amalgam was removed. At first it was replaced by a tested plastic, which itself was going to be replaced for good by a tested dental material after the excretion of the amalgam. For a while, during the removal of the amalgam and immediately afterwards, the heart problems increased dramatically. Again the medical doctor could only find a few extra systoles. As a result of the intensive support of the amalgam excretion with bioresonance therapy, the problems gradually got less severe and disappeared altogether after six months. Since then the patient still has minor problems now and then when she has a cold, but these are negligible compared with her original problems and they disappear after a few bioresonance therapies.

Bioresonance therapy in veterinary medicine

It is also possible to treat animals successfully with bioresonance treatment. In most cases they heal very quickly if it is used properly. This illustrates very clearly that the success of bioresonance treatment is not based on a placebo effect, as uninformed critics sometimes suggest. Have you ever seen an animal that "believes" in its treatment?

Objective healing success in veterinary medicine

Bioresonance therapy can be used in small animals as well as in cattle.

1. Case study:

Two sterilised cats, Turtle and Persian, five and six years old, had suffered for years from a severe itchiness with scabby dermatitis and a red, inflamed skin when touched. The animals were "glowing" as it were. They had been on cortisone injections every fourteen days for three years, at several hospitals. Without their cortisone injections, they simply could not live.
The practitioner took samples of everything they came into contact with in the house where they lived (blankets, cleaning agents, washing liquids, curtains,

foods, etc.). With the resonance test an unambiguous food allergy against certain proteins and certain preservatives was established.
The cats were treated once with the allergy program against the food allergy.
Shortly after the therapy the situation of the animals changed abruptly. The scabby spots on the skin disappeared and so did the itchiness. The practitioner gave the owner a diet plan with natural foods. The cats no longer get tinned food. More than five months later, the two cats are "as new", as the owner says.

2. Case study:

A 7-year-old gelding could not walk properly because of pain in the hindquarters. The paralysis had appeared suddenly, without apparent reason, and it was impossible to exactly locate the centre of the pain.
Four years previously the animal had suffered from a similar problem and at that time it had been X-rayed without the reason being found. The paralysis had disappeared after seven weeks of box rest and subsequent leading around at a walk. This time the veterinarian prescribed a painkiller and rest. But the owners did not want to lose the use of their horse for that long and tried their luck with bioresonance treatment.
The horse got four therapies with four days in between each one. The therapy programs and the position of the electrodes was decided by resonance testing.
The first therapy was started with a basic program as tested to balance the energy and as a preparation for the main therapy. The main therapy consisted of programs against joint arthritis and lymphoedema. The electrodes were positioned at the axis of the head and neck, at the base of the neck and in the saddle area as appropriate.
At the second and third therapies, programs against acute tissue processes and bruises were applied. And in the fourth and final therapy, a program against chronic tissue processes was added.

After two weeks the horse was no longer lame and could be ridden as usual.

Therapy blocks can also be present in animals

By the way, therapy blocks can also appear in animals. As in people, they can be caused by allergens, antibiotics, bacteria, vaccinations, scars, moulds, metabolic disorders, old accidents, viruses or other interfering factors such as not keeping animals in their natural environment. Geopathic stresses are less common because animals still are sensitive enough to feel and thus avoid them.

How patients can contribute to the success of bioresonance therapy

What patients should pay attention to in bioresonance therapy

Your co-operation increases the chances of healing

All healing depends on the co-operation of the patient. By this I mean the support of healing processes by positive thoughts and attitudes. This is no different in bioresonance treatment. Part of healing is the will to be healed.

There are other things that can help:

- Before the examination the patient should have been in the waiting room for a short while so that physical or psychological stress cannot influence the test results and the success of the treatment negatively.
- During the therapy the patient should:
  – close his eyes and concentrate on the problem area,
  – pay attention to whether during the therapy there are any negative reactions in the body,
  – if they do occur to report them to the practitioner so that he can continue the therapy until these reactions are over,
  – not speak with the practitioner or other people in the room.
- After the therapy the patient should:
  – report to the practitioner whether any physical

or psychological reaction took place during the therapy because this could be a valuable indication of interference fields or other indications for further treatment,
- if possible, not do hard physical work,
- avoid strong stimuli and tasks requiring a lot of effort for the few days following treatment so that the healing processes can continue without disruption,
- not drink alcohol or stimulating drinks (including coffee) for a few hours,
- drink at least 1 1/2 litres of low mineral water on the day of the therapy and daily afterwards until the end of the therapy to promote the toxin excretion,
- absolutely must have a shower the day after bioresonance therapy because of the excretion of toxins through the skin.

What the patient can do to make bioresonance therapy more effective

Bioresonance therapy relieves the patient of the oscillations of stressing, interfering factors. It goes without saying that these oscillations should not be built up again immediately after the therapy. For this reason the patient should avoid these stresses during and after the therapy. These could, for example, be tested allergens, but also clock radios at the head-end of the bed, unbalanced diet, shortage of sleep as well as habits and attitudes that work against the goal of the therapy.

Take advice!

If something is not clear the patient should discuss it with his practitioner.

Your attitudes influence healing

As we mentioned before, a positive attitude is an important precondition for healing. Doubting the possibility of becoming healthy or doubting the treatment method or the treating practitioner can be inhibiting factors. An unhealthy way of life can make it harder to heal. Dietary and drinking habits, exercise, sleep-wake rhythm and so on should be oriented towards a healthy life style.

Diet

- The diet has to be individual and adapted to the specific situation of the patient. So-called "ideal" diets or computer diet programs do not consider the individual metabolism, the individual need for energy, possible food allergies, etc. In general it can be said that the diet should be as low as possible in isolated refined sugar and free of pork. This is the case not only for the well-known reasons (sugar is a mineral thief, pork goes off easily), but also because these foods can absolutely block the treatment. Sugar, and products containing sugar, inhibit the activity and reproduction of the intestinal bacterium, Escherichia coli, which is vital in the intestines in a certain quantity to stimulate the lymph vessels of the intestinal wall. If the numbers of these bacteria are too small as a consequence of constantly eating sugar, the body's immune system is paralysed by insufficient stimulation of the lymph vessels of the intestinal wall and pathogenic bacteria can settle in increasing numbers in the intestines. The structure of pork protein is similar to human protein therefore it can easily seep through the intestinal wall and reach the blood. However, because pork is often contaminated with toxins, these toxins, combined with the protein, can easily slip into the human body and cause inflammations and allergic reactions.

Therefore: avoid sugar and pork!

Drinking water

- If it is to be health-promoting, drinking water usually has to be treated. Although treated in the waterworks, it is still contaminated with harmful substances and is also low in energy. In the framework of bioresonance treatment it is often necessary to relieve the body of clinkers, i.e. the water has to bind itself with these clinkers and excrete them from the body. This is only possible if the water molecules are not already "occupied" with other substances, for example with the so-called inorganic minerals or with chemical residues. In practice, clinkers can only be excreted with low mineral water. In order to do this there are some proven methods that I have described in my book "Secret Water" (not yet available in English).

Skincare

- The skin has many tasks, – for bioresonance therapy the excretion function is particularly impor-tant. Therefore special attention has to be paid to skincare. Faulty skincare can severely interfere with the therapeutic effect. This applies particularly to paraffin (kerosene) and allergens contained in skincare products. Paraffin (an oil derivative) is used in nearly all skincare products as an ointment base. It is cheap and causes few reactions which is why paraffin-containing skincare products are often advertised as "hypo-allergenic" or natural materials. But paraffin covers the skin with a non-breathing fat layer. The skin cannot breath any-more, excreted toxins collect in the subcutaneous tissue and can cause or increase inflammations there. This has to be avoided, particularly during bioresonance treatment; the tailback of toxins and clinkers to be excreted can essentially interfere with the treatment. Therefore only skincare products free of paraffin should be used, and not only by neuro-dermatitis patients. Skincare products con-taining allergens can lead to subliminal allergen stress. Many consumers are aware of this and use natural products. Unfortunately these often contain parts of plants that the consumers can react allergically to, for example camomile or St. John's wort. If you buy skincare products you have to pay attention to potential allergising components.

Sleep

- Sleep serves to regenerate the organism. Geopathic and technical electromagnetic stress in the bedroom can influence the organism so severely that sleep is not at all restful and this can interfere with treatment. Therefore the bedroom should be free from geopathic and technical interference fields. You should also take care to have a natural sleeping pattern.

Exercise

- Exercise is the engine of life. Exercise stimulates all physical functions. The modern life style without much exercise not only slackens the muscles but also the organ functions. This has the contrary effect to what bioresonance therapy is trying to achieve: the restoration of normal organ functions. Therefore you can increase the effect of bioresonance therapy by paying attention to physical training. Adaptations to increased demands reinforce the whole organism.

Epilogue: Bioresonance therapy as the medicine of the future

In every day practice it has been shown in thousands of cases that bioresonance was able to heal even though conventional medicine could make no progress. How is this possible ?

Because bioresonance therapy includes causes and levels of treatment that conventional medicine does not know about or cannot include because of their scientific concept.

Information as a therapy principle

This includes, for example, the vast number of interfering factors that I have considered in this book, the control of biochemical processes by information and the elimination of disharmonious oscillations by inverting them. However, these factors are realities that are gaining prominence in the awareness of many scientists and practitioners. In the long run it will be impossible for medicine to shut out these new findings and experiences.

Bioresonance as a precondition for successful treatment

From my point of view, bioresonance treatment is not just a certain treatment method with a certain type of device but a general precondition for successful holistic treatment. Every therapeutic signal should go into resonance with the body in order to become effective. To me, bioresonance treatment is the treatment of the future. Dr. Franz Morell, E. Rasche, Hans Brügemann and many involved practitioners are the pioneers.

I hope that through this book you have gained a good overview of the possibilities of bioresonance therapy and I hope that understanding bioresonance treatment will contribute to its successful effect for you.

Glossary

Abstinence: avoidance or disconnection of a contact, for example with an allergen.

AC (alternating current): an electric current that changes its direction of flow with a certain fre-quency; for instance a 50 Hz alternating current is an electric current that changes its flow direction 50 times per second.

Acupuncture: form of treatment from ancient Chinese medicine.

Acupuncture meridians: flow circuit in which according to the theory of acupuncture the physical energy circulates; they represent function circuits of the human organism.

Acupuncture points: special points on the acupuncture meridians where the skin resistance is reduced; these points are pierced with thin needles to amplify or attenuate the flow of energy.

Agranulocytosis: a high-level decrease of a certain group of white blood bodies (leucocytes); allergic and toxic reactions to medicines with skin inflammations.

Allergen: a substance foreign to the body that triggers antibody production and allergen-antibody reactions (allergic reactions).

Allergosis: an illness caused by the allergen-antibody reaction.

Alveolus membrane: the skin of the air vesicles.

Amplitude: intensity (level) of oscillation.

Anergy: the lack of reaction of an organism to an allergen.

Antibiotics: medicines to fight infections.

Antigen: substance that is recognised by the body as being foreign and that can trigger an immune response.

Antibodies: the immunoglobulins, protein bodies, that are produced by certain cells of the immune system as an answer to an antigen (for instance, an allergen).

Basic system (also: Basic regulatory system): the connective tissue as a regulatory organ that extends through the whole body.

BICOM: therapy device of bioresonance treatment, abbreviation of BIo-COMmunication.
Bioresonance: resonance in living beings, see also Resonance.
Bioresonance therapy: treatment with ultra-fine body, or substance's own, oscillations according to the bioresonance principle.
Bronchia: the two main stems of the windpipe.
Bronchiae: the branching out of the two bronchia.
Bronchioles: the branching out of the bronchiae in the lung tissue.
Cell plasma: the basic plasma of the cell.
Chemotherapeutics: active agents that inhibit the growth of or kill pathogens.
Clinical ecology: medical field of expertise, central are allergies and toxifications from foods, food chemicals and environmental chemicals.
Colonic irrigation: water treatment of the intestine.
Constitution: the individual spiritual-psychological-physical wholeness of the human individual that can be caused by disposition or changed by environmental influences.
Control circuit: a closed, cybernetic system relatively stable against interference.
Conventional: agreed upon by convention.
Corpuscle: small bodies, for instance blood bodies; in Physics: particles.
Crohn's disease: see Regional enteritis.
Cybernetics: science of the control and regulation of devices and organisms (biocybernetics) by information.
Cursor: term from the computer industry, indicator.
Decoder-dermographics: diagnostic device to examine the reactions of the skin after a stimulus.
Dermatosclerosis: change in the connective tissue of the skin.
Dermatosis: any kind of pathologic skin change.
Desensitisation: release of the readiness to react.
Diagnosis: naming a clinical picture, clinical course.
Dosimeter: device for measuring a radiation doses.
Dowser: expert who can assess geopathic and electromagnetic stress.
Dysbacteria: disturbance of the balance of the intestinal bacterial flora.
Electrodes: metal plates etc. that are able to conduct a current.
Electrolytes: chemical substances (bases, acids, salts) the solutions of which can be separated by an electrical current.
Endocrine glands: hormonal glands, for example pituitary gland, adrenal gland, thyroid gland.
Excretion: discharge; toxic metabolic product that is discharged from the body by the excreting organs.

Field: the area in the environment of a source of electric or magnetic energy in which a measurable force exists. We can also call it radiation in the sense that electromagnetic fields are radiated from the source and that they have the characteristics of particle radiation (see also Photon).

Field, electric: a power field that is created by elementary particles with a positive or negative load. Through the movement of the elementary particles an additional magnetic field is created at the same time; we then speak of an electromagnetic power field.

Field, electromagnetic: a power field that is created by every electric current and that emits from it; it has an electrical and a magnetic component.

Field, magnetic: the power field connected to electric currents (magnetic field).

Five elements theory: theory within acupuncture according to which the meridians are part of groups and influence each other mutually.

Focal toxicosis: toxification in the sense of a general illness. Is created by the release of substances (for instance decomposition products of dental protein or inflammation substances) created in a body area far away from the focus.

Foetus: the fruit of the womb during its development in the womb, called this from day 85 onwards.

Frequency: the number of oscillations in one time-unit, for example in seconds.

Frequency spectrum: the individual frequencies of a signal.

Functional circuit: the connection of functions of central and peripheral organs of the human being by way of a control circuit.

Gamma spectrometer: device to measure gamma rays.

Geiger counter: device to prove quantitatively the presence of ionising particles or quantum.

Human medicine: medicine concerning human beings.

Hyperergy: the increased reaction answer of a sensitised tissue to triggering stimuli (= allergy in the narrow sense).

Hypergy: the decreased reaction answer of a sensitised tissue to triggering stimuli.

Hyperkinesis: increased spontaneous motility activity, also psychologically-caused motile unrest.

Hypoergy: synonymous with Hypergy.

Hypophysis: see Pituitary gland: Endocrinal gland.

Hyposensitisation: weakening of the allergic reaction readiness.

Hypothalamus: see Pineal gland: a part of the interbrain.

Hz, Hertz: the frequency of electromagnetic radiation in oscillations per second.

Immunoglobulin (abbr. Ig): antibodies of the specific defence.

Information: a message that can be pictured electromagnetically by a series of different frequencies and amplitudes; for instance wheat has different electromagnetic information to cat hair.

Intolerance: non-compliance with external harmful substances such as medication, foods, additives.

Inversion: the process of turning around, in bioresonance the mirror-image turning around, of electromagnetic oscillations

In-vitro test: a test executed in a laboratory (vitrum = glass).

In-vivo test: a test on the living being.

Ion: an atom that has lost or gained one or two electrons, so that it has an electric load and, chemically, is much more active than a neutral atom, in which positive and negative load are in balance.

Ionising: the change-over of neutral atoms to ions by rays that have the power to loosen electrons from their positions.

Kinesiology: method of diagnosis and therapy that works in the sense of acupuncture with muscles that are assigned to certain meridians.

Measuring technique, gridded: a measuring method developed by the naturopaths M. Keymer and A. Schwarze used in bioresonance therapy in which the reaction to a therapeutic impulse is measured.

Mediator (substance): substance that is being released as a consequence of an allergen-antibody reaction which affects the tissue.

Microwaves: that part of the electromagnetic spectrum that in frequency reaches from 500 million oscillations per second (500 MHz) up to the frequencies of visible light.

Molecule: smallest unit of matter that can take part in a chemical reaction.

MULTICOM: a therapy device of bioresonance therapy, uses oscillations of colours, precious stones, sounds, metals, etc..

Mycosis: an illness caused by moulds.

Neural therapy: a healing method that uses specific procaine injections to restore normal circumstances in interference fields.

Non-tolerance: synonymous with Intolerance.

Nosodes: a homeopathic remedy made from illness products, similar to vaccine.

Orthomolecular medicine: a form of therapy that uses the "right molecules" to influence, for instance, the mineral and vitamin balance.

Oscillation: space-time-periodic change of a balance in which energy or information is transported, but no mass; the oscillation is characterised by length, frequency and amplitude.

Parameter: identifying value.
Pathogen: illness-causing.
Pathological: ill.
Photon: light particle, in an electromagnetic field bearer of energy; depending on the point of view it is particle or energy.
Physiological: normal, healthy.
Phytotherapy: healing with plants.
Pineal gland: a part of the interbrain.
Pituitary gland: endocrinal gland.
Potential: value for the energy of a body in a power field.
Pseudo-allergy: over-sensitivity reaction with allergy-like symptoms but without involvement of the immune system.
Quantum: smallest possible unit of matter, energy, information, space and time.
Radiation: transport of energy and information by wave and particle radiation.
Radioactivity: see Ionising.
Regional enteritis (Crohn's disease): inflammation in most cases of the terminal segment of the small intestines.
Regulation: adaptation of an organism to environmental influences with the aim of keeping up the normal physical functions.
Resonance: is given, when periodically changing forces (for instance, electromagnetic oscillations) meet with a system that is able to resonate (for instance, a human being) and stimulate it to resonate with them; during this the energy of the oscillation is transferred optimally to the receiver.
Segment-electrogram: diagnostic record of energetic conditions of segments of the body, received by electrodes.
Secretion: secretion product of the body, for instance from wounds.
Sensitisation: the development of an answer of the defence system by an antigen in the form of antibody production.
Skin potential: energy in measured skin areas.
Spectrum, electromagnetic: a form of classifying electromagnetic fields on the basis of their oscillation frequencies; the electromagnetic spectrum is divided according to frequencies, usages and different areas.
Symptom: sign of illness.
Syndrome: a complex of symptoms.
Systemic: affecting the whole system, for instance the whole organism.
Thermography: method of diagnosis, picture of the heat radiation of a person.
Tinnitus: noise in the ear.

Toxification: poisoning, harmful effect of vegetable, animal, chemical, bacterial toxins (endo- and exotoxins) on an organism.
Toxin: poison.
Treatment: measures to heal an illness.
Ulcerative colitis: ulcerative mucous membrane inflammation of the large intestines.
VEGA-test: a bioenergetic test procedure.
Veterinary medicine: medicine concerning animals.
Voltmeter: device to measure electric fields.
Wave: see Oscillation.

Literature

Becker, Robert O.: Heilkraft und Gefahren der Elektrizität. Bern, München, Wien 1993.

Braun-von Gladiß, K.-H.: Ganzheitliche Medizin. Südergellersen 1991.

Calatin, Anne: Das hyperaktive Kind. München 1992.

Flade, Sigrid: Allergien natürlich behandeln. München 1992.

Fritsch, Manfred: Gefahrenherd Mikrowellenherd. München 1994.

KATALYSE e.V.: Umwelt-Lexikon. Köln 1988.

Keymer, Martin (Hrsg.): Bioresonanz- und Multiresonanz-Therapie. Heidelberg 1990.

Keymer, M., N. O. Schmedtmann und R. Will: Bioenergietherapie – Ein ganzheitliches Diagnose- und Behandlungskonzept. Wiesbaden 1996.

Kuhlmann, Dirk: Die Pilz-Invasion. Lürschau 1993.

Leibold, Gerhard: Gesunde Darmflora. Wiesbaden 1992.

Leibold, Gerhard: Vorsicht Lebensmittel!. Wiesbaden 1995.

Mackarness, Richard: Allergie gegen Nahrungsmittel und Chemikalien. Stuttgart 1982.

Markus, Harold H., und Hans Finck: Ich fühle mich krank und weiß nicht warum. München 1992.

Randolph, Theron G., und Ralph W. Moss: Allergien: Folgen von Umweltbelastung und Ernährung. Karlsruhe 1984.

Schumacher, Peter: Biophysikalische Therapie der Allergien. Stuttgart 1994.

Smith, Cyril W., und Simon Best: Electromagnetic Man. London 1990.

Will, Reinhold D.: Geheimnis Wasser. München 1993.